Trigger Point Therapy

Unlock Your Body's Healing Potential And Improve Your Health Through Self-Treatment To Get Long-Lasting Relief.

Michele L. Valdez

Introducing the exclusive and captivating world of Michele L. Valdez. Immerse yourself in the timeless elegance and creativity that defines our brand. Experience the unparalleled craftsmanship and attention to detail that sets us apart. Discover the essence of sophistication and style with our exquisite collection.

Table of Contents

Preface

Discover a life free from chronic pain, limited mobility, and the constant struggle of feeling like your body is hindering your potential. Say goodbye to limitations and embrace a life of boundless possibilities. Are you yearning for a comprehensive solution that not only alleviates discomfort but also empowers you to seize control of your physical well-being and unleash your body's inherent healing potential? Are you ready to embark on an extraordinary transformative journey? Discover the incredible power of *"Trigger Point Therapy: Unlock Your Body's Healing Potential And Improve Your Health Through Self-Treatment To Get Long-Lasting Relief."*

Unleash the Incredible Power That Lies Within You

Experience a life where pain becomes a distant memory, where every day unveils a renewed sense of freedom and energy. Introducing "Trigger Point Therapy" - the ultimate guide that goes beyond a mere book. It's your personal roadmap to rediscovering your body's true potential and embracing a life filled with boundless vitality and wellness. Prepare to be amazed as you delve into the captivating pages of this revolutionary guide. Brace yourself for a transformative journey of self-discovery and empowerment, where you will unlock the secrets of Trigger Point Therapy. With this powerful knowledge in your hands, you will conquer pain, elevate your physical well-being, and unlock the untapped potential of your body. Get ready to embark on an extraordinary adventure towards a healthier, more vibrant you.

Experience the Power of Holistic Wellness: Beyond Pain Relief

Introducing "Trigger Point Therapy" - the revolutionary approach that goes beyond just treating symptoms. Say goodbye to temporary relief and embrace a holistic path to wellness. By targeting the underlying causes of pain and dysfunction, this therapy unlocks the door to lasting healing and vitality. Experience the difference today! Immerse yourself in the perfect blend of ancient wisdom and cutting-edge science with our comprehensive guide. Discover the transformative power of Trigger Point Therapy as it seamlessly intertwines with mindfulness practices, breathwork techniques, and nutritional guidance. Experience a holistic approach that nurtures your body, mind, and spirit from deep within.

Unleash Your Potential with the Power of Knowledge

Discover the incredible power of knowledge with "Trigger Point Therapy" - the ultimate resource that empowers you to seize control of your health and well-being. Unleash the tools and insights you need to unlock a world of endless possibilities. Discover the profound insights into the intricate workings of pain, unlock the secrets of effective self-treatment methods, and unlock the potential for personalized wellness strategies. With this extraordinary book, you will seize the power to become the mastermind behind your own transformative healing journey. Experience the liberating sensation of breaking free from reliance on medications or invasive procedures. Embrace the boundless possibilities of self-care and self-empowerment, and bid farewell to limitations.

Embark on a Transformative Healing Experience

Discover the extraordinary power of "Trigger Point Therapy" - a revolutionary approach that acknowledges and embraces the distinctiveness of every body. No two bodies are alike, and with this cutting-edge therapy, we honor and address the unique needs and challenges of each individual. Experience the personalized care and transformative results that only "Trigger Point Therapy" can provide. Introducing the ultimate guide for those battling chronic pain conditions such as fibromyalgia, myofascial pain syndrome, or headaches. But that's not all - if you're someone who wants to take your physical performance and overall well-being to the next level, this book is for you too. Packed with personalized advice and real-life solutions, it's designed to meet you exactly where you are on your healing journey.

Experience the Power of Unity

Embrace the empowering journey of those who dare to defy pain and limitations, opting instead to reclaim their bodies and seize life on their own terms. Join the movement today! Experience the transformative power of "Trigger Point Therapy" and become part of a vibrant community of individuals who share your passion for holistic health, self-empowerment, and embracing life to its fullest potential. Join us on a transformative journey as we redefine the boundaries of what's possible and tap into the boundless potential that resides within each and every one of us.

Embark on Your Journey Today

Are you prepared to embark on an extraordinary voyage of healing, empowerment, and transformation? Are you prepared to bid farewell to the burdens of pain and restriction, and embrace a life filled with boundless energy and optimal health? Discover the transformative power of "Trigger Point Therapy" and unlock the door to a vibrant and revitalized future. Congratulations on acquiring your copy today and embarking on the journey to unlock the incredible healing potential of your body. Embark on a captivating journey where the realm of possibilities knows no bounds.

Introduction

Discover a life free from the burden of chronic pain! Are you yearning for a solution that offers relief without the need for invasive procedures or potentially harmful medications? Unleash the incredible potential of Trigger Point Therapy, the revolutionary technique that is revolutionizing lives across the globe.

Embark on an enlightening journey with the esteemed wellness guru, Michele L. Valdez, as she unveils the secrets of your body's intricate network of trigger points in this all-encompassing guide. Discover the extraordinary power of these minuscule tension knots, as they hold the key to unlocking unparalleled relief from persistent pain, stubborn stiffness, and relentless discomfort.

Unlock the secrets of Trigger Point Therapy with the expert guidance of Michele L. Valdez. With a wealth of knowledge and the latest research at her fingertips, she effortlessly demystifies this powerful technique, ensuring that anyone in search of long-lasting relief can easily access its benefits. Introducing the ultimate solution for all your bodily woes! Say goodbye to back pain, migraines, and muscle tightness with this extraordinary book. Packed with practical techniques and easy-to-follow exercises, it's your ticket to effectively targeting and releasing those pesky trigger points. Don't let discomfort hold you back any longer - unlock the secrets to a pain-free life today!

Discover the transformative power of Trigger Point Therapy—a remarkable journey towards holistic wellness and lasting relief from pain. Experience the transformative benefits of the healing power of touch and breath. Discover a profound sense of relaxation, vitality, and freedom in your body like never before. Experience the freedom to live a life of boundless energy and radiant well-being. Embrace a future where limitations are a thing of the past.

Unlock a world of possibilities as you step inside and prepare to be amazed. Brace yourself for an extraordinary journey where you'll uncover a treasure trove of captivating wonders. Prepare to be captivated by a myriad

- Discover the ultimate guide to effortlessly finding and effectively treating trigger points

- Discover the ultimate self-care practices to effortlessly maintain a blissful and pain-free lifestyle.

- Unlock the power of mind-body techniques to elevate your well-being to new heights!

- Discover the awe-inspiring success stories of real people who have witnessed incredible transformations through the power of Trigger Point Therapy.

Unleash your inner strength and seize the reins of your well-being, paving the way for a pain-free existence. Discover the transformative power of Trigger Point Therapy, the ultimate guide to unlocking a brighter, pain-free future. Whether you're a seasoned wellness enthusiast or just embarking on your healing journey, this comprehensive approach will be your trusted roadmap.

Discover the incredible life-changing benefits of Trigger Point Therapy that have already transformed the lives of millions. Experience the ultimate transformation as you bid farewell to discomfort and embrace a vibrant new era of energy and optimal health. Indulge your body with the pampering it truly deserves.

Chapter 1

Discover the fascinating world of Anatomy and Etiology.

Discover the incredible world of trigger factors that emerge within the myofascial system, specifically in the core of a muscle's stomach where the engine endplate gracefully enters (known as the main or central trigger points). Introducing the remarkable palpable nodules, nestled within the confines of the mighty muscle, ranging in size from a mere 2 to 10 millimeters. These extraordinary nodules have the ability to manifest themselves in various locations, appearing in practically any skeletal muscle throughout the entire body. Discover the hidden power of Trigger points in your torso. Discover the incredible truth: this mysterious condition can manifest in infants and children alike, yet its presence doesn't always lead to the emergence of painful symptoms. Introducing Trigger Points: The Culprits Behind Myofascial Pain Symptoms, Somatic Dysfunction, Mental Disturbance, and Limited Daily

Functionality!

Introducing Myofascial Pain Syndrome - the ultimate solution for identifying and alleviating local pain originating from smooth tissue. Experience the power of muscle tenderness relief with Trigger Points - those tiny, yet mighty, points of sensitivity, measuring just a few millimeters in diameter. Discover the magic as they work their wonders at multiple sites within your muscles and the fascia of muscle tissue.

Discover the causes behind Trigger points, where aging is often a key factor.

Experience the unfortunate consequences of a fall, stress, or delivery trauma with our injury treatment.

Are you tired of feeling sluggish and lacking energy? It's time to break free from the sedentary lifestyle that's holding you back. Studies show that a staggering 45% of men between the ages of 27 and 55 are not getting enough exercise. Don't let yourself be part of that statistic. Take charge of your health and start incorporating regular physical activity into your daily routine. Your body will thank you!

Introducing the Posture Perfect Solution! Say goodbye to bad posture with our revolutionary system. Our expertly designed program targets common issues like top and lower crossed patterns, swayback posture, telephone posture, and even cross-legged seated positions. Get ready to stand tall and feel confident with the Posture Perfect Solution!

Are you tired of muscle overuse and the resulting micro stress from weightlifting?

Introducing the Persistent Stress Solution: Say goodbye to anxiety, depression, and emotional stress trauma. Experience a life free from the burdens of stress with our revolutionary program.

Introducing our revolutionary solution to address your health concerns:

- Boost your nutrient levels with our specially formulated supplements, including vitamin C, vitamin D, vitamin B, folic acid, and iron.

- Say goodbye to sleepless nights with our effective remedy for sleep disturbances.

- Introducing the revolutionary solution for joint problems and hypermobility.

Discover the fascinating world of Trigger points classification.

Introducing the remarkable world of trigger points, where possibilities are endless! Prepare to be amazed as we delve into the captivating realm of Main/Central and Supplementary/Satellite Result in Points. Brace yourself for an extraordinary journey!

Introducing the incredible Major or Central Trigger points - the true masters of pain! These remarkable points have the power to unleash intense local pain with a touch of pressure, and even radiate their discomfort according to the renowned referred pain map. Prepare to be amazed! Discover the remarkable foundation of these exercises, centered within the core of the muscle belly.

Introducing   the   remarkable   phenomenon   of

Supplementary or Satellite Trigger points, which emerge as a direct response to the presence of central Trigger points within the surrounding muscles. Experience the incredible phenomenon of spontaneous withdrawal when the central Trigger point is healed. Witness the presence of these remarkable occurrences in the form of a cluster.

Experience the power of being active and the tranquility of being inactive. Embrace the hidden potential within you, waiting to be awakened. Discover the beauty of the latent, the untapped energy that lies beneath the surface. Unleash your true Unleash the Power of Points

Discover the incredible power of the Active Trigger Point - a point that holds the key to unlocking tenderness and unleashing a unique pain pattern when gently palpated. Introducing the remarkable phenomenon of central Trigger points, which are not only Active but also accompanied by the presence of satellite Trigger points. While not all satellite Trigger points may be Active, their potential cannot be overlooked. Discover the hidden power of Trigger points. Inactive Trigger points hold the potential to transform into Active ones when a provocative factor comes into play. Unleash the untapped energy within.

Discover the hidden potential within your body. Inactive or Latent Trigger points, like hidden treasures, can manifest themselves anywhere, waiting to be unlocked with just a touch. These points, reminiscent of gentle lumps under your fingertips, offer a unique sensation that is far from unpleasant. Experience the incredible power of muscle tightening.

Experience the ultimate relief with our revolutionary technique: Diffuse Trigger Points. Say goodbye to muscle tension and discomfort as our skilled therapists target those stubborn trigger points, releasing built-up tension and restoring balance to your body

Experience the common occurrence of severe postural deformity, where primary trigger points multiply and secondary trigger points respond in a mechanism known as diffuse.

Introducing the revolutionary Attachment! Unleash the Power of Points

Experience the emergence of unparalleled softness in the tendon-osseous junctions. Don't let degenerative procedures of the adjacent joint go untreated - they can sprout and cause further complications.

Ligamentous Induce Points - the revolutionary solution for targeted pain relief!

Discover the remarkable potential of ligaments to develop trigger points. Discover the incredible impact of Trigger points in the anterior longitudinal ligament of the backbone, causing potential throat instability. Discover the incredible healing power of targeted treatments for leg pain syndromes, such as ligament patellae and fibular security ligament. Experience the relief you deserve and say goodbye to discomfort. Trust in the effectiveness of our proven methods to restore your vitality and well-being.

Unraveling the Mysteries of Pathogenesis and Theories.

Discover the mysterious origins of Trigger points. Discover the captivating world of Trigger points with these enlightening books that delve into their development, sensitization, and manifestation. While many ideas have attempted to explain this phenomenon, only a select few have stood the test of time with substantial proof.

Experience the extraordinary relief of Trigger Point pain, expertly managed by the delicate balance of thin myelinated fibers and unmyelinated fibers. Experience a wide range of stimulating and invigorating events, from mechanical triggers to chemical mediators. These occurrences have the power to awaken and heighten the responsiveness of A fibers and C fibers, playing a crucial role in the formation of Trigger points.

Introducing the groundbreaking Integrated Result in Point Hypothesis (ITPH) - the cutting-edge working hypothesis of our time. Experience the fascinating world of sarcomeres and electric motor endplate. Discover the intricate interplay of these dynamic elements that can lead to remarkable pathological changes at the cellular level. Uncover the secrets behind their overactivity, driven by a multitude of intriguing factors. Brace yourself for a journey into the captivating realm of mobile pathology. Experience the transformation of these sarcomeres, leading to a powerful inflammatory response, a decrease in oxygen and essential nutrients, involuntary shortening of muscle fibers, and an intensified metabolic demand on local cells. Experience the captivating world of electrophysiological investigations of Trigger points, where fascinating phenomena unfold. Delve into the realm where electrical activity emanates from dysfunctional extrafusal engine endplates, rather than from ordinary muscle spindles. Prepare to be amazed!

Introducing the remarkable polymodal theory, a groundbreaking explanation for the presence of polymodal receptors (PMRs) that span across your entire body. These extraordinary receptors, when exposed to specific unrelenting or pathological stimuli, transform into powerful induce points.

Introducing the groundbreaking Radiculopathy theory! This revolutionary concept unveils the direct correlation between nerve root issues and the emergence of both local and distant neurovascular indicators. Prepare to be amazed as we delve into the fascinating world of Trigger point creation!

Discover the fascinating world of Peripheral and Central Sensitization. Uncover the secrets behind chronic or amplified pain by exploring the intriguing trends of both central and peripheral sensitization. Prepare to be amazed! Experience the undeniable phenomenon of central sensitization, triggered by an intense or repetitive stimulus of the nociceptor in the periphery. Witness a remarkable surge in excitability and synaptic effectiveness of primary nociceptive pathway neurons, all of which can be reversed. Experience the extraordinary sensation of heightened sensitivity to pain, known as tactile allodynia and hyperalgesia, which is triggered by even the slightest touch or pressure. Discover the remarkable CNS changes that can be identified through cutting-edge electrophysiological or imaging techniques.

Discover the Power of Differential Diagnosis

Introducing Fibromyalgia - the condition characterized by a pervasive sense of fatigue and discomfort that permeates the entire body. Experience a world where joint pain is a thing of the past. Our revolutionary solution is designed specifically for women, targeting not only the joints but also the muscles, bones, tendons, ligaments, and even body fat. Say goodbye to discomfort and hello to relief with our innovative formula that targets those tender points. Introducing Soft Factors: Discover discrete regions of tenderness nestled within gentle cells, delivering a localized sensation of pain. These areas are exquisitely sensitive to the gentle touch, yet patients do not exhibit any outward signs of discomfort or follow any known pain patterns. Discover the intriguing world where these two pain syndromes intertwine, their symptoms overlapping in a mysterious dance. Only through a thorough examination by a seasoned physician can the veil be lifted, revealing the true nature of these enigmatic conditions. It is even possible that they are not separate entities at all, but rather interconnected forces, working in harmony to challenge the boundaries of our understanding.

Introducing the incredible impact of muscle pain! Prepare

to be amazed as we unveil the hidden truth behind this discomfort. Brace yourself for a revelation: muscle pain can be caused by a variety of conditions, including the notorious musculoskeletal diseases. Yes, you heard it right! These conditions can lead to muscle pain, leaving you longing for relief. But fear not, for we are here to guide you on your journey towards a pain-free life. Say goodbye to muscle pain and embrace a future filled with vitality and well-being!

- Introducing the revolutionary solution for occupational myalgias!

- Introducing the revolutionary Post-Traumatic Hyperirritability Syndrome solution!

- Introducing the revolutionary solution for joint dysfunction - osteoarthritis. Say goodbye to discomfort and hello to a life of freedom and mobility.

- Introducing the perfect solution for those pesky tendonitis and bursitis woes.

- Experience the cutting-edge world of neurological disorders.

- Introducing Trigeminal Neuralgia: The Ultimate Solution for Pain Relief!

- Introducing Glossopharyngeal Neuralgia: The Ultimate Guide.

- Introducing the remarkable Sphenopalatine Neuralgia!

- Introducing: Systemic Diseases - The Silent Threat

- Introducing the remarkable systemic lupus erythematosus (SLE) - a condition like no other.

- Introducing the revolutionary solution for Rheumatoid arthritis.

- Introducing Gout: The Ultimate Solution for Joint Pain!

- Introducing Psoriatic Arthritis: The Perfect Blend of Beauty and Pain Relief.

- Introducing a comprehensive range of health concerns that we address with utmost care and expertise: • Unleashing the power to combat infections, be it viral, bacterial, protozoan, parasitic, or Candidiasis infection. • Tackling the notorious Lyme disease head-on, with our cutting-edge solutions.

- Introducing the perfect solution for those dealing with the challenges of hypoglycemia and hypothyroidism. Say goodbye to the struggles and hello to a healthier, more balanced life.

- Introducing: Heterotopic pain of central origin!

- Introducing Axis II-type disorders - the next level of psychological conditions.

- Introducing the extraordinary phenomenon of psychogenic pain.

- Introducing: Painful Behaviors - the ultimate solution to your discomfort.

Discover the telltale signs and remarkable clinical

findings.

Are you tired of living with chronic pain conditions? Say goodbye to headaches, pains everywhere, early morning stiffness, TMJ symptoms, tinnitus, and more. It's time to address the root cause of your discomfort - the active bring-about point. Let us help you find relief and reclaim your life.

Experience the Transformation of Flexibility (ROM)

Experience the occasional discomfort of movements and activities that may intensify symptoms. Experience the discomfort of tension headaches, migraines, ringing in the ears, and temporomandibular joint problems? These symptoms are often associated with these conditions. Discover the fascinating world of postural abnormalities and their remarkable compensations.

Discover the Power of Diagnostic Procedures

Discover the cutting-edge world of Trigger point diagnosis, where no lab test or imaging technique has yet been established. Unlock the mysteries of this fascinating field and explore the possibilities that lie ahead.

Introducing Anamnesis: The Key to Unlocking Your Clinical Background Discover the truth about fibromyalgia and its presence in your family's medical history. Uncover the secrets hidden within your genes. Discover the power of understanding an individual's physical and day-to-day activities. By delving into their existence, we can uncover valuable insights. It's important to inquire about their exercise habits and level of activity, as a sedentary lifestyle can potentially be a pathogenic factor. Discover the hidden factors that could be impacting your well-being. Delve into the world of (chronic) muscle overuse, daily stress, medications (and their overuse), and sleep disruptions. Uncover the truth by asking the right questions and analyzing every detail.

Discover the Power of Examination

Discover the art of pinpointing the exact location and activating the perfect trigger point. Discover the key to unlocking optimal muscle health: identifying nodules, whether big or small, and lumps that may appear individually or in clusters within the muscles and fascia. Keep an eye out for any noticeable changes in temperature or relaxation of the skin, indicating the presence of active trigger points. Your journey to improved well-being starts with recognizing these vital signs. Discover the key indications to ensure that we are in the right place: • Experience the initial onset of pain and the subsequent recurrence, both originating from muscular sources.

Introducing the incredible phenomenon of reproducible spot tenderness! Experience the sensation of muscle tenderness right at the location of the Trigger point pain. But that's not all - brace yourself for the mind-blowing effect of pain being referred locally or even far away with just a simple mechanical activation of the Trigger point. Prepare to be amazed! Experience the familiar discomfort and sensitivity that arise from the unique features of this muscle, faithfully recreating the area of concern for the patient.

Experience the persistent relief you've been searching for with our revolutionary solution. Say goodbye to muscle stiffness and embrace the freedom of a relaxed body. Our innovative technology targets the palpable hardening of tight muscle fibers, providing a soothing sensation that will leave you feeling rejuvenated. Imagine a tender spot transformed into a harmonious symphony, as the shortened muscle unwinds like the strings of a finely tuned guitar. Discover the power of our breakthrough treatment today.

Experience the incredible sensation of a taut flesh responding with a captivating twitch, as a leap of excitement occurs when the activation point is stimulated.

Experience the convenience and versatility of conducting examinations through palpation in various positions - whether standing, seated, or prone. Introducing the essential components of a comprehensive assessment: the ROM exam and postural evaluation. These crucial steps must not be overlooked.

Introducing the Power of Outcome Measures

Introducing Fischer's groundbreaking solution: the pressure threshold meter (algometer). This innovative tool not only allows for the precise measurement of Trigger points, but also provides a quantitative record of the effects of physical therapy treatment. Say goodbye to guesswork and hello to accurate documentation. Discover the incredible results of the analyzed tests, where pressure pain threshold and visible analogue level (VAS) ratings took center stage as the key measures. Discover the power of ROM, the ultimate tool for analyzing therapy results.

Experience the power of Medical Management with our cutting-edge approach. Discover the transformative benefits of our carefully curated selection of Medications. Experience the soothing relief you deserve with our selection of over-the-counter medications. Say goodbye to mild pain with the powerful combination of Tylenol (acetaminophen) and non-steroidal anti-inflammatory drugs (NSAIDs) like aspirin, ibuprofen, and naproxen. Trust in our trusted remedies to bring you the comfort you need. Experience relief from muscle pains and stiffness with the powerful combination of acetaminophen and NSAIDs. Not only do they effectively decrease pain, but NSAIDs also work to reduce swelling, providing you with relief from inflammation and discomfort. When over-the-counter drugs fail to bring relief, turn to the expertise of a healthcare provider. They may prescribe a range of effective solutions, including muscle relaxants, anti-anxiety drugs like Valium, antidepressants such as Cymbalta, or NSAIDs like Celebrex. In some cases, a short-term course of stronger painkillers like codeine, hydrocodone, and acetaminophen (Vicodin) may be recommended. Trust in the power of professional guidance to help you find the relief you deserve.

Introducing the revolutionary Point Injection (TPI) procedure, where a tiny needle is skillfully inserted into the patient's Active Trigger point. Experience the cutting-edge treatment that brings relief like never before. Experience the ultimate pain relief with our revolutionary injection. This powerful solution combines the soothing effects of a local anesthetic or saline with the added benefits of a potent corticosteroid. Say goodbye to discomfort and hello to instant relief. Experience the power of our revolutionary infusion technique that effortlessly renders trigger points inactive, providing unparalleled relief from pain. Discover the incredible power of a short treatment that can bring you long-lasting relief. Experience the convenience and efficiency of receiving shots from your trusted physician. With a quick and seamless process, you'll be in and out in no time. Experience the convenience of visiting multiple sites in just one click. Experience an innovative solution for allergic reactions to medication with our dry-needle technique. Say goodbye to the worry of adverse drug effects as we offer a drug-free approach to address your specific needs.

Experience the transformative power of Physical Therapy Management.

Introducing the revolutionary Trigger points! Say goodbye to everyday-life factors that cause discomfort. Our innovative solution eliminates or reduces these triggers, allowing you to live your best life. But that's not all - we also provide position training and education on postures and lifestyle, ensuring you maintain optimal health and well-being. Experience the difference today!

Introducing the revolutionary techniques of Passive Extending and Foam Roller Extending! Experience the incredible benefits of these methods, performed just a few times each day. And that's not all - indulge in the luxurious practice of Self-Massage, a ritual to be enjoyed multiple times per day. For the ultimate relaxation and rejuvenation, don't miss out on the Deep Stroking Therapeutic Massage, expertly executed in a rhythmic and unidirectional manner. Elevate your wellness routine today!

Introducing our revolutionary strengthening program: starting with the power of isometric exercises and progressing to the dynamic intensity of isotonic exercises.

Introducing the Ischemic Compression Technique: a groundbreaking treatment that harnesses the power of ischemia to target and alleviate trigger points. By applying consistent pressure, this technique induces ischemia in the trigger point zone, providing effective relief. Discover the intriguing theory that challenges conventional wisdom. Delve into the fascinating world of Trigger points and their mysterious nucleus, which is said to harbor a remarkable condition known as hypoxia. Uncover the secrets that lie within this enigmatic phenomenon. Introducing Simons' revolutionary treatment modality - a game-changer in the world of Trigger point therapy. Say goodbye to the unnecessary induction of additional ischemia in the Trigger point area with Simons' Trigger point Pressure Release. Experience the power of this cutting-edge technique without any hassle or discomfort. Experience the revolutionary system designed to liberate contracted sarcomeres within the Trigger point. Experience the perfect balance of pressure as it gently eases away tension and strain within the Trigger point area. Our expert technique ensures a gradual and soothing relaxation, without any discomfort. Discover the art of precise pressure for ultimate relief. Witness remarkable progress in range of motion with both of these techniques after treatment.

Introducing the Revolutionary Taping Technique!

Experience the power of the Spray and Extend Technique

with ethyl chloride application. Unleash the benefits of Manual Lymphatic Drainage (MLD) as it works to overcome the obstacles caused by trigger points, allowing for optimal lymphatic flow.

Introducing the incredible world of proprioceptive neuromuscular techniques! Prepare to be amazed by the transformative powers of Reciprocal Inhibition (RI), Post-Isometric Relaxation (PIR), Contract-Relax/Hold-Relax (CRHR), and Contract-Relax/Antagonist Contract (CRAC). These cutting-edge techniques are designed to unlock your body's full potential and enhance your overall well-being. Say goodbye to limitations and hello to a new level of physical excellence!

Introducing a range of specialized techniques to enhance your well-being. Experience the transformative power of Neuromuscular Technique (NMT), Muscle Energy Technique (MET), and Myotherapy (MT). Our state-of-the-art facilities also offer cutting-edge treatments such as Ultrasonography, Hot and Chilly packages, Diathermy-Tecar therapy, Laser beam, and Ionophoresis. Discover the ultimate in therapeutic care.

Introducing the all-new, revolutionary concept of "Other Managements"! Experience a whole new level of efficiency, effectiveness, and innovation with our cutting-edge approach.

Discover a world of potential therapies waiting to be unlocked within the pages of books.

Introducing a wide range of captivating themes for your consideration. Please note that while these themes are undeniably intriguing, it's important to acknowledge that not all of them boast concrete scientific evidence. Explore with an open mind and let your imagination soar! Discover the fascinating world of studies, where the power of placebo effects can't be ignored. While most studies may not be placebo-controlled, it's important to consider the possibility of immediate results after treatment. Dive into the realm of scientific exploration and uncover the hidden truths behind these intriguing phenomena.

Introducing our cutting-edge treatments for pain relief and rejuvenation: • Experience the transformative power of Dry Needling, a technique that targets trigger points to release tension and promote healing. • Discover the ancient art of Acupuncture, a holistic approach that stimulates the body's natural healing abilities and restores balance. • Unleash the healing potential of Laser therapy, a non-invasive treatment that uses light energy to reduce pain and inflammation. • Explore the innovative Prolotherapy, a solution-based therapy that injects carefully selected substances around trigger points to alleviate discomfort and promote tissue regeneration. Say goodbye to pain and hello to a life of vitality with our range of advanced therapies.

Advantages of Induce Point Treatment

The benefits of induce point treatment, which is an optional therapy, center on identifying and releasing trigger points. Located in the skeletal muscle, these trigger points hurt when squeezed. Trigger points often develop as a result of damage to the muscle fibers.

Trigger point therapy, sometimes referred to as myofascial trigger point therapy or neuromuscular therapy, is primarily used to treat pain-related problems. Activate points can be released using a variety of methods, including as dry needling, therapeutic massage, and chiropractic adjustments.

Induced Point Therapy Applications

Trigger point therapy is used in alternative medicine to treat a variety of chronic pain issues, such as low back pain, temporomandibular joint pain, and headaches.

In addition, a lot of people utilize trigger point treatment to treat sports injuries, tinnitus, migraines, osteoarthritis, and carpal tunnel syndrome.

Compared to Traditional Acupuncture, Induce Point Therapy

Dried-out needling is a popular type of trigger point therapy that entails putting a needle (without medicine or injection) into the affected area. It is important to distinguish between dry needling and acupuncture, which is a form of traditional Chinese medicine in which needles are used to stimulate points believed to be connected to routes that distribute vital energy, or "chi," throughout the body.

The primary goal of trigger point therapy is not to increase chi circulation because there are certain similarities that result in point sites and acupuncture point sites. Moreover, activation point treatment is generally used to treat musculoskeletal ailments, whereas acupuncture can be used to treat a wide range of health issues.

Back Ache

For those with persistent low back pain, dry needling may be helpful when used in addition to other therapy. That is the conclusion of the 2005 study that was published in the Organized Reviews Cochrane Data source. However, the authors of the review note that additional research is required to fully understand the effectiveness of dry needling in treating low back pain, as the majority of the investigated studies were of low quality.

Headaches

According to research, trigger point therapy can be used to treat tension headaches. This is in line with a 2012 Expert Overview of Neurotherapeutics study. Unfortunately, there weren't enough research trials to evaluate the use of trigger point therapy for treating tension headaches.

Pain in the Heels

A 2011 study that appeared in the Journal of Orthopaedic and Sports Physical Therapy reveals that point therapy outcomes can help reduce plantar heel discomfort.

Sixty individuals with plantar heel plan were divided into two groups for the analysis: While the other group received trigger point therapy in addition to the same stretching regimen as the first group, one group engaged in regular stretching exercises. The group who had the point therapy outcome showed a more notable improvement in physical function and a more notable decrease in pain after a month.

Parkinson's illness

Pilot studies that were published in Movement Disorders in 2006 indicate that trigger point therapy is certain to alleviate certain Parkinson's disease symptoms.

Thirty-six Parkinson's patients who either had music-based rest therapy or trigger point therapy twice a week were included in the analysis. Users of the bring about point therapy group showed a more notable improvement in engine operation by the end of the trial. Though the quality of life increased somewhat in both groups, only the individuals in the music rest group saw changes in their emotional state and level of anxiety.

Methods for Applying Trigger Point Repair

If trigger point therapy is something you're considering, consult a physician for guidance on locating a qualified provider.

It's too soon to declare activation point therapy a cure for almost any ailment because to the paucity of studies. It's important to keep in mind that postponing or avoiding conventional treatment and self-treating disorders can both have detrimental consequences. Make sure to speak with a physician before utilizing induce point treatment for any kind of medical condition.

Chapter 2

Advantages of Point-Based Therapy

It is believed that activated point therapy blocks the brain signals that result in pain and results in a point. The goal is to both alleviate discomfort and retrain the muscles to function without it. In this manner, neuromuscular pain's tightness and inflammation are lessened, flexibility is raised, and coordination and versatility are enhanced. Additionally, the therapy helps lower blood pressure and enhance blood flow.

Trigger point therapy can be used to treat a variety of conditions, such as tendinitis, arthritis, carpal tunnel syndrome, headaches, menstrual cramps, multiple sclerosis, muscle spasms, stress and weak points, sciatica, temporomandibular joint symptoms (TMJ), tendinitis, and whiplash accidents.

Generally, a member of the medical community refers to a person who does trigger point therapy. A brief history of any unintentional injuries, jobs had, and sports participation will be required by the therapist. She or he will ask the designated person to go into great detail about the kind and location of the pain.

The coordinating trigger point's area will be probed by the therapist. It is possible to achieve this by probing with a dried-out needle or by injecting lidocaine, saline, or other drugs. After the point is available, the therapist will apply painful pressure for a few seconds utilizing their fingertips, knuckles, or elbows in myotherapy.

Treatment is frequently felt right away. After applying pressure or administering an injection, the therapist will gently stretch the muscles in the bring-about point. Lastly, a customized set of exercises is taught to the patient in order to retrain the muscles and prevent further pain.

Workbooks are available so that patients can treat themselves at home to get the most out of trigger point therapy.

Getting Ready

Before starting active point therapy, people should consult a medical professional to make sure that their pain isn't being caused by a disease or fracture. An accredited induce point therapist will not treat a patient who is not referred to them by a medical expert.

Usually, the patient receives therapy on a padded table or chair. The typical individual should dress comfortably and loosely. Facilitating the classes will be an ongoing, open dialogue with the therapist.

Thirty to an hour can pass between treatment sessions. Approximately $45 to $60 is spent on each program. It is possible to ease acute suffering with multiple applications. Treatments for chronic pain may need to be multiple.

Take Care

People who have recently been in an accident or have infectious disorders should wait to start point therapy until they have fully healed.

After starting point treatment, people on prescription anticoagulant medicines may have bruises.

Studies and Widespread Adoption

Even if a few recently published studies of activation point therapy have been linked to the increased acceptance of acupuncture within the mainstream medical establishment. Induce point therapy is becoming more and more popular in Europe, Asia, and America. A recent study conducted by a number of Japanese specialists found that outcome in point treatment was superior than conventional allopathic medications in terms of alleviating the pain associated with renal colic.

According to the American Academy of Pain Management (AAPM), studies on the effects of trigger point therapy on headaches and back pain have only involved groups of fewer than ten participants. Nonetheless, the AAPM introduces point treatment as a legitimate approach to pain management and alleviation.

Trigger point therapy can be thought of in the original medical profession as an adjunct to treatment. Many medical researchers, including psychiatrists, orthopedic cosmetic surgeons, and anesthesiologists, are familiar with their patients.

The Operation of Trigger Point Therapy

A number of factors can cause trigger points to appear, including postural stress from standing or sitting incorrectly for extended periods of time at a computer, psychological anxiety, stress, allergies, dietary deficiencies, irritation, and dangerous toxins in the environment. Muscle stress can also result from repetitive motions during play or from automobile accidents, falls, sports activities, and work-related accidental injuries, among other things. A single incident can initiate a trigger point, and if it is not managed appropriately, you could pay the price for any future ones you may have.

Reasons for Pain

Your instinct is your body's attempt to protect itself after a damaging "event". It can accomplish this by changing your posture, gait, and sitting or standing position, which puts uneven strain on your bones, tendons, ligaments, and muscles. This results in muscular imbalances related to strength and versatility as well as postural dysfunctions in your body.

If this were sufficient, your blood flow may become restricted. When this happens, your peripheral and central nervous systems will start to send out those "referred" pain signals, which will complicate diagnosis and therapy. For this reason, some experts believe that Induces points will mark the beginning of the fibromyalgia process. Is there much more that might go wrong? Continue reading.

Here's a great example of how a single trigger point in a muscle can result in sciatica, back pain, or a herniated disc to help explain the process. The most typical location for a trigger point is the Quadratus Lumborum (QL), a region of the low back that is located just above your hips. Your QL will gradually become dysfunctional—that is, it will tighten and shorten as you limit its use—no matter what kind of incident sets off the Trigger point.

As the QL becomes more and more dysfunctional, the pelvis will shift in alignment. When the pelvis degenerates, the backbone is forced into an atypical curve, which unevenly strains the disc. The disk will begin to swell over time. This example, within your general standard of living, will progressively worsen. Depression frequently follows.

Finding Your Inducement Points

All people have "activate" variables. The question is: You are extremely likely experiencing the effects of an induce point if you have persistent pain, tightness, or difficulty doing certain movements. Dizziness, earaches, sinusitis, nausea, acid reflux, false heart pain, cardiovascular arrhythmia, genital pain, and numbness in the hands and feet are just a few of the symptoms that can be brought on by trigger factors.

Headaches, jaw and neck discomfort, low back pain, sciatica, lateral epicondylitis, carpal tunnel syndrome—you name it—can all be brought on by trigger points. They will be the means of obtaining joint discomfort that is commonly misdiagnosed as arthritis, tendonitis, bursitis, or ligament injury in the wrist, hip, leg, and ankle joints. If you think this is too much, you should read Dr. Greg Fors' book "Why We Harm: an entire Physical & Religious Guide to Recover from Your Chronic Pain," in which he explains the fundamental cause of a wide range of ailments.

Here are a few additional signs to be aware of: You have TPs if you experience any of the following symptoms: uncomfortable menstruation, irritable intestine symptoms, toothaches, exercise plateaus, restless leg syndrome, etc.

A single person's cells cannot be altered by just applying heat, vibrating massagers, or massage lotion to the top layer of the epidermis. Sufficient and continuous deep pressure must be applied to the "knotted-up area." The body will experience soft tissue release as you work the trigger point, which will promote improved blood flow, a reduction in muscular spasm, and the disintegration of new scar tissue. It will assist in clearing out any accumulation of toxic metabolic waste.

Additionally, the body will experience a neurological release that will lessen pain signals to the brain and reset your neuromuscular system to resume normal function. In other words, everything will function as it should once more.

Looking for Solace

The duration of your trigger point experience is one of the criteria that determines how long it takes to release a trigger point. The number of activation elements you possess, the efficacy of your current treatment, and the frequency at which you may give or receive treatment are additional factors.

If you are lucky enough to find a doctor who can accurately assess your condition—let alone treat induce points—it might still take a lot of time and money to compensate you for fully releasing all of the main, latent, and myofascial result in points that you may possess. You can try seeing a therapeutic massage therapist, however trigger points need to be addressed on a daily basis using a method that will apply the required identity pressure because they are very erratic. It will probably not be feasible to see a therapeutic massage therapist often enough to receive a trigger point release.

A Sense-Based Approach

The Main Concept Is Simple

First of all, a trigger point is the size of a mustard seed, which is among the smallest seeds. The idea is to regularly subject the area to prolonged strain for a certain amount of time. You can use a number of different methods that are available to accomplish this. As a result, you'll need to give it some thought.

"There is no replacement for understanding how to control your musculoskeletal pain," according to Dr. Simons. "Dealing with myofascial trigger factors yourself addresses the foundation of this kind of common pain, and it is not only a way of temporarily reducing it." In other words, you are far more adept than anybody else at fixing your own activate points—once and for all. Dr. Simons is precisely correct when he says that you must stay knowledgeable about your issue and then put what you've learned into practice. This contradicts the conventional wisdom of today, which holds that if we are sick, we should find you to take care of the issue on our behalf.

Taking Charge of Your Care

Naturally, there may come a time when you will want medical assistance. On the other hand, you will be treated better the more you know. That will typically take some time and effort on your behalf, but the benefits will accrue more quickly and yield superior outcomes.

Counsel

To be sure the issue isn't considerably worse, first consult your doctor. Many physicians now recognize the value of massage therapy and may write a prescription for it, allowing you to use your insurance or flexible spending account to pay for the service.

Chapter 3

Where Can I Find the Answer Regarding the Area Around My Neck?

Mechanical causes—that is, those that impose tension or strain on muscle tissue—are typically the cause of trigger points. Trigger points can be caused by a spinal injury, such as whiplash from a car accident or an injury sustained during sports.

By performing daily activities that are repetitious and detrimental to the health of your spine over time, you can even promote the development of a trigger point. For example, carrying a large handbag that puts tension on your neck, spine, and shoulders, or sleeping with an unsupportive pillow or craning your neck while using a computer are two ways that you can cause strain to your neck muscles.

Are Trigger Factors and Fibromyalgia Tender Factors the same thing?

Many times, trigger sites are mistaken for fibromyalgia's

soft components. Though they won't be the same, bring about points and sensitive elements are both isolated areas of discomfort.

Referred pain or pain that spreads is not caused by tender circumstances; rather, they are the catalyst for such pain. Soft variables associated with fibromyalgia are likewise symmetrical, appearing on both sides of your body. Asymmetrical designs do not exhibit trigger considerations.

But this is where things become tricky: Individuals with fibromyalgia may experience both trigger points and tender spots. It is common for those who have fibromyalgia to also experience symptoms of myofascial pain. In those cases, it's critical to discuss with your physician the specific methods for managing those various types of pain.

Why is it difficult to diagnose trigger factors?

Although trigger factors are frequently the cause of many different types of spine pain, from low back pain to throat pain, doctors still don't know a lot about them. Physicians are not familiar with the process by which trigger factors result in visible pain, nor do they have a standard criteria for bringing about points.

Complex trigger factors include: Both of these are simple to identify but challenging to diagnose. They have the ability to directly cause muscular soreness, which may be easy to see. They can, however, mirror other issues, which makes them difficult to find. Fibromyalgia and myofascial pain symptoms are frequently mistaken for one another. A trigger point in the throat could be the cause of persistent jaw discomfort, earaches, or toothaches.

Consult a physician about the possibility of activate factors being the source of your persistent throat pain if you don't know what is causing it. Your doctor might refer you to a physiatrist or other specialist in the backbone to check for potential causes in your throat, shoulders, and spine.

"Pulling the Trigger": The precise management of Myofascial Pain Syndrome and Trigger Factors

Myofascial pain syndrome and trigger factors can be treated with anything from simple home remedies to injections that your doctor has to provide. As the medical profession continues to research the symptoms of myofascial pain, no one "magically" cures myofascial pain. To locate a remedy, you might wish to look into a few possibilities.

In-Home Treatments

You should start using an at-home remedy right away if the trigger point discomfort is too much for you to handle. To properly address the issue, you need first consult a trained professional, such as your doctor, a therapeutic massage therapist, or a physical therapist, to determine where the problem is located. Only then can you start home therapy.

The typical method of treating trigger points is massage, which might be difficult if they're located close to your spine in an awkward spot. If you are unable to reach the area with your hands, rolling over a baseball or rugby ball gently and slowly can provide immediate relief.

Massage treatment

Deep tissue massage may relieve an irritating trigger point. Qualified massage therapists are trained to relieve muscle pain. Regular therapeutic massage sessions can help lessen the occurrence of myofascial pain symptoms and persistent trigger points.

Although the precise mechanism by which dry needling reduces activation point pain is unknown, treatment entails injecting a bright needle and moving it around. Blood flow to the induce point muscle region is thought to be encouraged by this therapy, which may lessen muscular contraction. In the vicinity of the point location, this therapy may also help inhibit pain signals, however further research is needed to validate this.

Physical Medicine

Physical therapists can use ultrasound, electric stimulation, heat, massage, and other techniques to treat trigger points. In order to relax and lessen the tensed muscle, they could also apply a cooling spray to the area around the bring-about point before performing focused extensions.

Drugs

Various muscle relaxants have been employed to mitigate the symptoms associated with myofascial pain. Since they frequently cause sedation or other side effects, their usage should be restricted and should only be combined with a first-rate physical treatment regimen. Drugs like Valium (diazepam) should be avoided since they might cause addiction and induce drowsiness.

Initiate Point Subjections

Your doctor might suggest trigger point injections if you have symptoms of myofascial pain and, even after attempting the aforementioned therapies, you continue to experience recurring trigger factors. These injections are thought to be a later stage of healing for trigger points; in other words, your doctor could advise you to attempt less intrusive therapies like therapeutic massage therapy before switching to injectable therapy. For optimal comfort and effectiveness, your doctor might also recommend that you combine your injections with a physical therapy or exercise regimen. These should not be administered repeatedly, and injectables should not contain steroid drugs. Usually, all that is needed for these shots to effectively reduce pain and promote improved rehabilitation is a simple saline injection mixed with a small amount of Novocaine (procaine).

Factors that Trigger the Throat: "Knot" as Clearly Defined as You Thought

Most people have had a good couple of muscular around our throats, but when it comes to diagnosis and therapy, these spots are best left unseen. You can help avoid contributing factors and symptoms of myofascial pain by practicing excellent posture and maintaining healthy vertebral technicians. Having access to various therapies, such as physical therapy and therapeutic massage, can help prevent chronic pain from interfering with your daily activities if you suffer from it.

Chapter 4

Where Can I Find the Answer Regarding the Area Around My Neck?

Mechanical causes—that is, those that impose tension or strain on muscle tissue—are typically the cause of trigger points. Trigger points can be caused by a spinal injury, such as whiplash from a car accident or an injury sustained during sports.

By performing daily activities that are repetitious and detrimental to the health of your spine over time, you can even promote the development of a trigger point. For example, carrying a large handbag that puts tension on your neck, spine, and shoulders, or sleeping with an unsupportive pillow or craning your neck while using a computer are two ways that you can cause strain to your neck muscles.

Can we compare fibromyalgia trigger factors to fibromyalgia tender factors?

Many times, trigger sites are mistaken for fibromyalgia's

soft components. Though they won't be the same, bring about points and sensitive elements are both isolated areas of discomfort.

Referred pain or pain that spreads is not caused by tender circumstances; rather, they are the catalyst for such pain. Soft variables associated with fibromyalgia are likewise symmetrical, appearing on both sides of your body. Asymmetrical designs do not exhibit trigger considerations.

But this is where things become tricky: Individuals with fibromyalgia may experience both trigger points and tender spots. It is common for those who have fibromyalgia to also experience symptoms of myofascial pain. In those cases, it's critical to discuss with your physician the specific methods for managing those various types of pain.

Why is it difficult to diagnose trigger factors?

Although trigger factors are frequently the cause of many different types of spine pain, from low back pain to throat pain, doctors still don't know a lot about them. Physicians are not familiar with the process by which trigger factors result in visible pain, nor do they have a standard criteria for bringing about points.

Complex trigger factors include: Both of these are simple to identify but challenging to diagnose. They have the ability to directly cause muscular soreness, which may be easy to see. They can, however, mirror other issues, which makes them difficult to find. Fibromyalgia and myofascial pain symptoms are frequently mistaken for one another. A trigger point in the throat could be the cause of persistent jaw discomfort, earaches, or toothaches.

Consult a physician about the possibility of activate factors being the source of your persistent throat pain if you don't know what is causing it. Your doctor might refer you to a physiatrist or other specialist in the backbone to check for potential causes in your throat, shoulders, and spine.

"Pulling the Trigger": The precise management of Myofascial Pain Syndrome and Trigger Factors

Myofascial pain syndrome and trigger factors can be treated with anything from simple home remedies to injections that your doctor has to provide. As the medical profession continues to research the symptoms of myofascial pain, no one "magically" cures myofascial pain. To locate a remedy, you might wish to look into a few possibilities.

In-Home Treatments

You should start using an at-home remedy right away if the trigger point discomfort is too much for you to handle. To properly address the issue, you need first consult a trained professional, such as your doctor, a therapeutic massage therapist, or a physical therapist, to determine where the problem is located. Only then can you start home therapy.

The typical method of treating trigger points is massage, which might be difficult if they're located close to your spine in an awkward spot. If you are unable to reach the area with your hands, rolling over a baseball or rugby ball gently and slowly can provide immediate relief.

Massage treatment

Deep tissue massage may relieve an irritating trigger point. Qualified massage therapists are trained to relieve muscle pain. Regular therapeutic massage sessions can help lessen the occurrence of myofascial pain symptoms and persistent trigger points.

Necessary Care

The precise mechanism by which dry needling reduces activation point pain is unknown to experts, but it entails injecting a bright needle and moving it around. Blood flow to the induce point muscle region is thought to be encouraged by this therapy, which may lessen muscular contraction. In the vicinity of the point location, this therapy may also help inhibit pain signals, however further research is needed to validate this.

Physical Medicine

Physical therapists can use ultrasound, electric stimulation, heat, massage, and other techniques to treat trigger points. In order to relax and lessen the tensed muscle, they could also apply a cooling spray to the area around the bring-about point before performing focused extensions.

Drugs

Various muscle relaxants have been employed to mitigate the symptoms associated with myofascial pain. Since they frequently cause sedation or other side effects, their usage should be restricted and should only be combined with a first-rate physical treatment regimen. Drugs like Valium (diazepam) should be avoided since they might cause addiction and induce drowsiness.

Initiate Point Subjections

Your doctor might suggest trigger point injections if you have symptoms of myofascial pain and, even after attempting the aforementioned therapies, you continue to experience recurring trigger factors. These injections are thought to be a later stage of healing for trigger points; in other words, your doctor could advise you to attempt less intrusive therapies like therapeutic massage therapy before switching to injectable therapy. For optimal comfort and effectiveness, your doctor might also recommend that you combine your injections with a physical therapy or exercise regimen. These should not be administered repeatedly, and injectables should not contain steroid drugs. Usually, all that is needed for these shots to effectively reduce pain and promote improved rehabilitation is a simple saline injection mixed with a small amount of Novocaine (procaine).

Factors that Trigger the Throat: "Knot" as Clearly Defined as You Thought

Most people have had a good couple of muscular around our throats, but when it comes to diagnosis and therapy, these spots are best left unseen. You can help avoid contributing factors and symptoms of myofascial pain by practicing excellent posture and maintaining healthy vertebral technicians. Having access to various therapies, such as physical therapy and therapeutic massage, can help prevent chronic pain from interfering with your daily activities if you suffer from it.

Chapter 5

Relieve Throat, Upper Back, Spinal Cord, and Other Pain with Therapeutic Massage.

The cantankerous scalene muscle group is located privately of the throat, deep within the Anatomical Bermuda Triangle. While working in this ethereal region, therapeutic massage therapists have disappeared, never to be seen again. Because the area and its muscles are unique and complex, many therapeutic massage therapists with less training are hesitant to work with it. This brief article describes how various joint pain issues in the neck, chest, arms, and spine can involve the scalene muscles and how to massage the scalenes to relieve pain in these locations. Although challenging to use, the scalenes are a rewarding muscle group!

A cartoon featuring a man and a medical professional

A sword is lodged in the man's throat. But according to

the caption, "It's my hands." "My hands hurt," is an example of the uncommon pain that might be associated with the scalenes.

"Doctor, it's my hands. My hands ache.

The muscle group called scalenes is peculiar. You might want to start with my advanced throat pain tutorial if your pain is severe or unrelenting.

Headaches and collective throat pain are often associated with the scalenes, but that's only the top of the iceberg. This is an isolated region, to be sure: compared to other torso muscular tissue, the scalenes frequently have more varied and unusual trigger points. Pain in the scalenes is commonly felt almost anywhere, however the scalenes themselves are the primary system affected by this oddity. The sensation of "known pain" It could hurt your upper body instead of your scalenes.

Observed pain effects are typical of all muscle pain or any other type of inner pain; for example, shoulder and equip are affected by cardiac episodes; nonetheless, the scalene muscles frequently produce remarkably complicated, modifiable, and significant patterns of pain that are well-known. The outcomes can be a little strange, causing symptoms that many people—including physicians and therapists—never would have thought were caused by the scalenes.

Diagram displaying the pain-producing areas identified by the scalene muscle group. This diagram illustrates how scalenes may be involved with discomfort in the upper body, spine, jaw, face, headaches, equip, and hands.

Causing Suffering

The pain from sore scalene muscles travels throughout the upper body, spine, hands, hook, and medial side of the top, much like the pain from a heart attack spreads from the center into the glenohumeral joint and arm. The discomfort felt in the trunk could be likened as a sharp agony that pierces the torso.

Furthermore, other "interesting" (in the sense of the Chinese language curse) effects of scalene trigger sites include those on your voice tone, swallowing, emotions, and feelings that permeate your entire mind, as well as your sinuses, hearing, and teeth. Scalene Trigger points, in my experience, are clinically highly relevant to disorders that don't seem to be related, like:

- A singer who performs professionally but whose tone seems to be mysteriously declining (release of the scalene and other trigger points in the throat helps)

- At least two patients with bothersome, severe chronic sinus infections had surgery in an attempt to treat the condition (one patient was nearly treated by scalene activation point release alone, while the other one only received minor relief).

- Having a number of patients with severe cases of what I refer to as "brick back again," a condition in which the area between your shoulder blades feels like a cinder block instead of bone and muscle because it is so rigid and imprisoned.

- Because tight scalenes can impinge on the brachial artery and brachial nerve plexus in the neck, they can cut off the circulation and neurological supply to the equip.

- the "Globus sensation," which is the feeling of a lump in the throat in the absence of a real mass.

Therefore, stimuli that cause scalene are "episode queens," exhibiting symptoms and results that are disproportionately large for such small and hidden muscles. They frequently have a part in other mishaps that affect the entire area. Scalene Trigger points have the same potential to ruin an area as gangs. It is clear that the anterior scalene causes problems; it both causes and exacerbates a wide range of other issues.

The Scalene Religion

Could it be that the clinical necessity of scalenes has been overstated? Many therapeutic massage therapists place some body muscles on an odd pedestal and use them as the scapegoat for an excessive number of disorders. The psoas muscle, a huge muscle tucked down deep in the stomach and pelvis, is the classic example of muscle mystique; however, the scalenes are perhaps the other prime example, as they are physically identical.

Traditional Grey

Along with other deep throat flexors, the scalenes

Psoas buzz is plain absurd; it has very little substance, and my "Perfect Places" series purposefully omits it. But there's a more substantial kernel of truth in scalenes buzzes. Yes, many experts overstate the importance of scalenes; nevertheless, there is a slightly more sensible explanation for this than there has been in the past.

The deep anterior muscles of the cervical spine, which include the scalenes, form a more considerable band of deep cervical flexors. To treat sore throats, it's rather common to try working these muscles. Refer to Deep Cervical Flexor Training: "Primary" throat conditioning.

The Anatomical Bermuda Triangle's Anatomy

To contribute to the ribs above the collarbone, the scalenes fan out straight from the sides of the neck bone pieces. The anterior, middle, and posterior scalenes are the three muscles that make up the scalene group. They frequently apply pressure to the topmost borders of the neck vertebrae and the bottommost upper ribs. As a result, the scalenes mostly drag the head laterally with their minds. Furthermore, because of the way they pull through to the ribs, they are breathing and exhaling muscles even though they are moving the throat.

Here's something even more strange that adds to the intrigue surrounding this muscle group: in certain people, the scalene muscles extend between the ribs and attach directly to the highest point of the lungs; in many others, they even extend between the bones and attach to the highest point of the lungs. Other than the diaphragm, these are the only muscles that attach directly to the lungs. They penetrate to the membrane known as the pleura, which contracts to enclose the lungs. Quite the odd muscle group! In actuality, this kind of anatomical heterogeneity is rather common across all of our anatomy.

As an organization, the scalenes are not difficult to locate, but their features are detailed. They occupy the space created by the triangle's three apparent constructions:

The Bone

The lengthy V-shaped throat muscles (sternocleidomastoid, or, if that seems like too much mouthwork, just the SCM) and your shoulder muscles (trapezius)

Where are the scalene muscle group and optimum spot No. 4?

The location of Perfect Place 4 is within the triangle. I don't want to take you on a wild goose chase after trying to locate the exact spot, but there is undoubtedly one specific region, in the stomach of the center scalene, that I believe is the most usual clinically significant result in point. Patients are likely to feel important in this location. You should investigate all possible locations within the triangle, as they may prove to be relevant. Additionally, things change: Perfect Place 4 might keep one section of the triangle intact one day and another section elsewhere. It's not necessary to treat oneself precisely; it's vital to be open to modest experimentation.

As a helper, the best way to approach this area is from above, with the recipient facing up. It is beneficial to place his or her concentration on the bed's portion in the absence of a therapeutic massage table. Keep your fingers smooth and position the pads of your fingertips in the triangle's hollow: above the collarbone, in front of the large trapezius muscle and its maximum length, and outside the prominent neck muscles that form the V-shape of the sternocleidomastoid muscles.

The hands will be in this position, slightly bent inward and pointing roughly toward the sternum. Now apply moderately firm pressure, using finger pads rather than fingers, both downward and slightly inward on the ropy muscles that encircle the triangle. You may activate some trigger points and tense muscles by using a lot of power, and you never have to worry about being too precise.

Using your fingertips, softly strumming across the ropy rings of muscles, explore the triangle by making little circles. The area is rich in opportunities to bring about points, some of which will be worthwhile and fascinating.

Danger!

This location is somewhat vulnerable if you do

something dumb; there is a chance that you could pierce arteries or nerves. Generally speaking, avoid giving this area a strong massage and, out of compassion, avoid using any instruments here.

The pulse is visible if you do touch the jugular vein or carotid artery; calm down. It's not a nice place to rub. You no longer feel the need to massage your carotid artery rather than your eye. Nerves are incredibly robust and can withstand much more pressure than most people know, thus smaller vessels are not an issue, although it could be risky to take chances in this field.

Exist anything more? Although the voice box and trachea are sensitive, they are also too central to obstruct the therapeutic massage of the scalene, and no one would put unwarranted pressure there.

What Kind of Therapeutic Massage Should Scalene Offer?

Certain muscles respond better to massage than others. Generally speaking, therapeutic massage is not enjoyable for the scalene. The throat is a vulnerable area of the body. People are becoming more and more afraid of pressure, so don't underestimate it. This is especially true if you don't know that therapeutic massage is safe or don't recognize the strange emotions that are so prevalent in this area. A really mild method may feel a touch hot, nasty, and questionable at first—not the kind of Trigger point you want to play about with for fun, as it seems that fragility translates into sensitivity. Whoa, give me a hint! It sounds great, doesn't it? It's not all terrible news, though.

Some people find that scalene massage is enjoyable straight out of the package, while others may need some time to "work through" and become accustomed to the more unpleasant sensations. The best-case scenario, though, is when you are resolving an issue. For example, if your scalenes are stressed out and causing chronic pain, this will feel like you finally finding the spot where you could never reach to scratch an itchy spot.

To increase your chances of having a good experience, massage the scalenes with broader, less "poky" pressure while working gently and with respect. The best-case scenario from such pressure is more likely to be a strange deep pain that spreads to the chest, back, mind, and arms. The wonderful suggestion patterns make the scalenes feel essential, the focal point of the spot. At its best, scalene therapeutic massage appears tough yet "serious." When a whole limb "lamps up" and becomes visibly painful due to a slight pressure in the throat, many individuals will say something along the lines of, "What the hell is going on?"No muscle generates more astounding remarks than this one. Many may say something along the lines of, "Holy, what the actual hell is that? "when they see a whole limb "lighting up" and clearly hurt from a slight pressure in the throat.The scalenes may be painful and unpleasant to massage at first, but this Perfect Place can be quite effective in the long term. That is generally true of most known pain, and it is similarly true of all Perfect Areas, but "some activate factors are more the same than others."

Thus, relax and be ready for anything.

Though it's probably true that in order to reach the better feelings, you need to "sort out" a small amount of unpleasantness. Don't be cruel in this field; "no pain, no gain" does not apply here. It takes time for patients to adjust and "accept" the enthusiasm in this sector. Respectfully persevere, and there's a good probability that the sensation will shift from hot to warm and from sharp to achier. It might switch over in five minutes, or it can require a few days of diplomatic maneuvering with the area. There is, however, a reasonable amount that you should try to achieve. This Perfect Place isn't that perfect, and you should ignore it, if after a reasonable amount of time your time and effort don't start to show signs of improvement.

The earliest known cause of lateral epicondylitis was tennis, although there are other causes as well.

The relationship between breathing (theoretical but conceivable)

Inefficient breathing in and out may be a contributing factor in a number of joint aches and pains, especially in the upper back, neck, and shoulders. Though this is simply a theory, the relationship between discomfort and disordered breathing is rooted in a fundamental idea: when the diaphragm isn't functioning properly, the pectoralis small and the sternocleidomastoid and scalene muscles in the neck try to take over. Sadly, these muscles aren't designed for regular breathing, and they can strain to the point of discomfort and injury. A range of uncomfortable chest muscle issues could arise, from garden variety tightness to comparatively unlikely but serious repercussions including whiplash, rotator cuff injuries, and thoracic store symptoms.

In this case, the muscles that are most likely to produce symptoms are the odd, irritable scalenes. Start by looking at the Respiration Connection to learn more.

The relationship

The rule that, if it exists, ties the relationship between discomfort and dysfunctional inhalation and exhalation is as follows: the pectoralis minimal and the sternocleidomastoid and scalene muscles in the throat attempt to take over when the diaphragm fails to do its duty. Unfortunately, these muscles wear out and eventually hurt themselves because they aren't designed for program respiration.

Anything that makes breathing more difficult could easily lead to excessive scalene usage. While there are many possibilities, smoking is perhaps the most common and avoidable—it also happens to be a risk factor for chronic pain on its own, so it's a double-edged sword. Although this is just conjecture, smokers' item respiratory muscles cannot only contain a disproportionately higher number of trigger elements, but also more unpleasant, persistent, and nastiness.

A Startling Connection between Lateral Epicondylitis and Your Scalenes

This connection between lateral epicondylitis and other disorders is a great example of how peculiar and clinically relevant the scalene is, typically to conditions that initially seem unrelated.

A condition known as "lateral epicondylitis," or lateral epicondylitis, affects a lot of racquet sports players and typists. The scalene muscle group is crucial to this condition. Although it is typically described as an inflammatory illness, things are rarely that simple. Regardless of lateral epicondylitis, it's likely that myofascial trigger points, specifically Perfect Place No. 5 in the forearm muscles, have a significant impact.

Furthermore, it appears that Perfect Place No. 4 has a big influence on Perfect Place No. 5. Trigger factors on the forearm trunk are described as "scalene muscle induce points are generally the main element to [treatment of] forearm extensor digitorum result in points" by Travell and Simons. Thus, there is an intriguing advantage to treating Perfect Place No.

Chapter 6

Simple Ways to Do Self-Massage for Myofascial Pain in Points.

Learn how to release your own trigger points, or knots in your muscles. It may seem as pointless to massage oneself as it does to desire to tease oneself. When there are valid reasons to massage your muscles, though, the culprit is most often muscular "knots" or trigger points, which are sensitive little patches of clenched muscle fibers that hurt and feel tight. They may play a major role in a number of common pain issues, such as throat and low back pain. Most minor trigger points can probably be resolved on their own.

Self-massage could help you sleep better than a massage therapist in situations like this. While specialized assistance might be beneficial and even necessary in certain cases, identifying ways to prevent trigger factors may also be more economical. It is a reasonable, affordable, and safe self-help technique for the majority of common pain issues.

It's also a contentious one:

- There is sufficient scientific disagreement regarding trigger elements. It's true that mammals experience discomfort in some sensitive areas of our smooth tissue, but little is known about their personalities, and the widely held belief that they resemble tiny cranks may not be accurate. We're not even sure if massaging them is effective. One potential experimental pain treatment is trigger point massage.

- The fundamental ideas behind using self-massage to treat trigger points are explained in this educational essay. For a more in-depth look into the topic, check out my extensive guide on myofascial pain and activators.

For what reason are few trigger points easy to manage?

An inexpensive golf ball or your thumbs can be used for very basic self-massage, which can relieve a great deal of trigger point pain. Even though trigger elements can be really unpleasant, most of them are easy to locate and eliminate with a little massage.

It sounds too good to be true, but according to Dr. Janet Travell, "nearly every treatment" can alleviate a condition to some extent, and self-massage is typically the simplest, least expensive, safest, and most effective. Thus, we ought to be skeptical about it. How do these pointless treatments operate?

It's possible that the pain becomes more of a sensory phantom than a sign of a tissue problem. With therapeutic massage, it can be easier to improve because there isn't much to "fix"—just a feeling that needs to get better.

For minor muscle knots, self-massage alone is usually the most effective treatment. But how can these insignificant remedies function?

Alternatively, like stirring a sauce until lumps disappear, it's possible that the massaging really increases muscle mass directly. It's possible that therapeutic massage functions by pushing waste products and their metabolites out of the bring-about point, potentially breaking a vicious cycle and keeping the trigger point from reoccurring. But no one has had the chance to show what kind of muscular "knot" may be released by therapeutic massage up until now.

It is probably much easier to control isolated trigger sites because they are neurologically easier to understand. There is far more probability of success if the issue is limited to one bodily component.

Simple Guide to Self-Massage for Trigger Points

For a straightforward situation, only a few mild massages may be sufficient. A few days' worth of bigger dosages of massage—just a few minutes—will probably be sufficient for moderate cases. The most difficult cases that can be treated at home might require spending about six five-minute sessions per day for a week. But none of these are grounded in research, and therapy will always fall short.

Here are a few fundamental pointers:

With what rub? Use your fingers, thumbs, fist, elbow, or

whatever appears most comfortable and available to you to rub the activation spot. Easy-to-reach places benefit from simple instruments; these include different balls and other handy things. Remarkably nourishing is the therapeutic massage with a golf ball! Of course, using a foam roller would be beneficial, but for most tasks, the contact area is too large.

A tool like the Backnobber from Pressure Positive can be important. But there are other quick and simple self-massage tools around the house that are almost as effective as a tennis ball!

How should one rub? For simplicity, simply press straight down on the induce-point, hold it for a short while (10–100 seconds), or use tiny circular or backward and forward kneading motions without worrying about the direction of the muscle fibers. Everything is fair game. On the other hand, stroke parallel to the tissues as though you wish to elongate them because that could be more successful if someone happens to learn the way of the muscle fibers, which is occasionally obvious.

How hard is it, Rub? There are more difficulties with this! Since the main goal of therapeutic massage is to have a conversation with your nervous system, you should purchase to have the authority to strengthen: kind and supportive! Not awful or impolite. The process should have a strength that is Goldilocks-perfect—that is, robust enough to meet needs while being manageable. Please aim for the 4–7 range on a scale of 1–10, where 1 is painless and 10 is excruciating. Err on the side of gentleness at first. Newbies are usually far too passionate. (As well as the experts!)

How should it feel exactly? In general, pressure applied to the muscle knot should be distinct, strong, and satisfying; it should have a calming, pleasant effect. "Good pain" is what that is. A therapeutic massage is an opportunity to talk to your nervous system.

It also implies that you want the proper sculpt for it. Kind and supportive! Not awful or impolite. You most likely need to be more gentle if you're gritting your teeth or wincing. You ought to be able to unwind. For additional information on what a therapeutic massage that produces results should feel like, see the next section.

What if things goes wrong? Most likely, not if the demand is reasonable. On the other hand, let go if you experience any unfavorable reaction in the hours following therapy. With essential therapy, you may count on cells to adjust over the course of a few days of consistent treatment to stronger demands. If they don't, then either bring-about points aren't the issue or these are (much) worse trigger variables than you initially believed.

Where to rub? You may rely on your instincts for simple self-care: massage the area that hurts! While it is important to search for sensitive areas, you can focus your investigation on a manageable portion of the muscle around the "epicenter" of your symptoms. For instance, look for trigger variables primarily in the finest of your make if your glenohumeral joint hurts. (Don't worry too much about this; you won't always be able to feel a lump or "knot" in your muscle.)

What if the discomfort is not at the activate point?

introduce elements that could cause symptoms to arise elsewhere than at the site of induction. What should a novice do? This is the main outcome of point treatment, so don't worry about it too much. Keep in mind that known discomfort may be misinterpreted, but don't worry about it until your vital therapy isn't working.

How much rub is that? For around thirty seconds, give or take depending on how beneficial it feels, give each suspected trigger point a therapeutic massage. For the majority of trigger factors, this is sufficient—especially if you think you have multiple that require attention! There is no limit to the amount of time that can be spent on any trigger point; if you find that repeatedly massaging it makes you feel good, feel free to continue. Five minutes is about the maximum that each trigger point will require at one time.

Rub, how frequently? You should therapeutically massage any body point that seems to need it at least twice a day, or up to half a dozen times a day, provided you are not having any negative reactions. More is probably simply going to get annoying too quickly and be too likely to merely irritate it.

How can you tell whether it is effective? When a trigger is obtained, a tiny representation of the thumb pressing downward on the myofascial trigger point signifies "release." To achieve a "release," self-massage for trigger points is used. What exactly is a "release" at this stage, and how does it feel? How are you going to define success? It mostly denotes a loosening of consciousness regarding the trigger point and a softer tissue texture—the knot melting.

But the word "release" is ambiguous and lacks a precise scientific definition. It's a term for the unknown, for whatever is undoubtedly happening when the final appearance of the Trigger point disappears. Perhaps it marks the actual rest (or possibly the violent disruption!) of the tightly knotted muscle fibers. Alternately, it might be "just" a sensory version, which would only cause temporary pain and require some recuperation (like itching a mosquito bite).

There may not be a clear release. Before things get better,

they might even feel worse: after a current discharge, cells may continue to be "polluted" by waste products and their metabolites. One possibility is that the release could necessitate some damage to the muscle knots' tissue. If so, even after you've succeeded, the area is probably highly sensitive.

It's an odd mix of possibilities where both are treating and being treated: first, there's a satisfying yet deep sensation of scratching an itch, but the tissue is actually more sensitive afterward, not less.

For novices, don't worry about the details: engage the trigger point, have faith that you have most likely achieved a release, even if it's only partial, and wait for the trigger to show that you are calm. If you were successful, you would see a reduction in symptoms quickly—usually by the next morning.

If you were successful, you would see a reduction in symptoms quickly—usually by the next morning. Pleasant discomfort? When natural induce factors are involved, a successful release is usually linked to "good pain"—a distinct, powerful, and satisfying sensation that is simultaneously painful and relieving. It is beneficial in the same way as puking is beneficial: although it is unpleasant, the body "knows" that it needs and desires a great deal of pressure. In most cases, a trigger point release is far more likely if you experience "good pain."

On the other hand, you almost definitely need to be kinder if you are gritting your teeth or wincing. For many patients, comfort can be a crucial component of a successful course of treatment! You're too hard on yourself, especially in the beginning, if you can't massage the outcome in point constructively without crying. A trigger point may occasionally feel unpleasant, hot, and burning, yet it may still release. But frequently, addressing a bad trigger point like this calls for more intensive or long-term care. Remarkably complex is the "pressure question" of how much is too much.

The Trigger point is only the tip of the iceberg.

There are several reasons why simple self-massage techniques might not work. The doubters might be correct; perhaps the only thing present is an odd feeling and nothing that can be fixed in the body. Alternatively, it could fail for very technical reasons: the trigger point might not be located in the same location as the pain due to the neurological phenomena known as "referred pain." The only way to stop this from leading people astray and rubbing it in the wrong places is via experimentation and education. More options exist in a similar vein, especially for more constrained circumstances. This explains why I wrote a self-help book about myofascial pain in its entirety.

Has Your Neck Been Knotted?

You could strumming a guitar with the muscles in your neck. But this song is definitely not pleasant to listen to. Is the aching muscles you're rubbing, pressing, and prodding really getting better? Or would you be aggravating the situation?

Your stiff muscles might start to whistle a more cheerful melody by following a few simple steps. Chad Adams, DC, a chiropractor, explains the subtleties of trigger point massage:

An exaggerated response to muscular knots

Muscle knots are those ropy, taut threads in your throat and those kinks in your back again. They may be regions where muscle tissue has tensed up and refused to release; they are also known as trigger points.

A muscle spasm, according to Dr. Adams, is a notice from the mind that something is wrong and that the person is about to panic and become tense. Trigger factors establish a pattern of recurring actions. That might be like repeatedly swinging a rugby racquet or, for most people, stooped over our desks and tapping away at the keyboard all day.

"Your body can withstand a lot of stress, but humans weren't designed to perform the same task repeatedly, every day," he asserts. "Those are calls for help from those few places."

Thus, how can the muscles that are tense be relaxed? According to Dr. Adams, self-massaging the bring-about points by pressing on the muscle knots is an excellent place to start. Stress from nature might aid in muscle relaxation.

This is how self-massage is done:

- Locate the confined spaces (you probably won't need to search far).

- Firmly push into the trigger points with your fingertips or with equipment like foam rollers and therapeutic massage balls.

Ideally, repeat three to five minutes each time, or five or six times a day. According to Dr. Adams, "it requires participating in the day-to-day routine."

How challenging is the event you lead? It fluctuates. Some people are built to withstand tremendous pressure, while others—no shame—are a little more sensitive. Go ahead and get started; Dr. Adams believes it's unlikely that you'll exert enough pressure to cause any harm.

However, it couldn't feel wonderful right away. "The area of the process is pain," he says. Severe pain is not, though. If you experience a sharp pinch or tingling, you probably have a non-muscular personal injury. If such is the case, stop using your thumbs immediately and see a doctor. Remain persistent: Make a big adjustment to your surroundings

Each mini-massage should leave the muscles feeling more relaxed. Regular trigger point massages can assist provide longer-lasting relief as time goes on.

But think about other things you may change around you to improve the quality of your muscle tissue as well. Would a more comfortable desk chair improve your position? Is it feasible to prolong breaks throughout the day?

If after making those adjustments the knots still come back for more, it might be time to call in the experts. Think about consulting a professional such as a physical therapist, chiropractor, or therapeutic massage therapist.

Chapter 7

What Illness is Causing My Persistent Throat Pain?

Numerous problems frequently cause discomfort in the neck. Furthermore, pain throughout the neurological pathways may cause problems in the head, hands, equip, and glenohumeral joint. The legs and the region beneath the throat may become inflamed due to spinal cord pain.

Numerous Throat Conditions

The majority of neck pain instances resolve in a few days or weeks, but discomfort that lasts longer than a few weeks may indicate a serious medical issue that needs to be treated. For the best outcomes in some cases, early intervention can be necessary.

Picking Out Symptoms of Neck Pain

The following symptoms can be similar to throat pain:

- The stiff neck, which makes it challenging to turn the top.

- A single point of stabbing or razor-sharp pain.

- Tenderness or soreness throughout the body.

- Pain that travels up into the head or into the arms, fingertips, or shoulder blades.

- Sometimes the neck pain is accompanied by additional symptoms that are even worse, such tingling, numbness, or weakness that travels to the hands, fingers, or shoulder.

- Having difficulty holding or lifting objects.

- Problems with balance, coordination, or walking.

- Intestinal or bladder dysregulation.

When Does a Tight Throat Become Serious?

The guitar neck ache could be little and easily overlooked, or it could be so severe that it prevents you from doing basic daily tasks like sleeping. The pain may be transient, intermittent, or persistent. If unidentified, throat pain could potentially indicate a serious underlying medical condition like meningitis or cancer.

A strain or sprain is one type of personal injury that can exacerbate cervical spine issues.

What Could Go Wrong with the Cervical Backbone?

The amazing task of supporting and allowing mobility for the top, which may weigh up to 11 pounds—roughly the same as a medium bowling ball—falls on the neck, or cervical spine.

Throat Pain Treatment

The majority of throat pains can be managed non-surgically, at home with self-care, and with guidance from a medical professional.

Self-Care for Throat discomfort:

Generally, neck discomfort that is not incapacitating and did not originate from trauma can be managed by the patient on their own. Among the self-care strategies for throat pain are:

- *Calm down:* For the majority of throat sprains and strains, resting is sufficient for a few days, since the tendons and muscles heal on their own. It's critical to use caution to stay away from strenuous activities or movements that exacerbate existing pain.

- **Warmth and ice:** Using snow as an anti-inflammatory may help reduce pain and inflammation. Applying glaciers or cold packs to throat pain initially is simpler since they can temporarily constrict tiny arteries and stop discomfort from getting worse. Once a few days have passed, temperature or snow can be used alternately. Increased inflammation may result from continuous high heat application.

- **Massage:** A therapeutic massage helps relieve muscle tension and spasms, hence reducing discomfort. It is commonly used after administering glaciers or warmth.

- **Improved posture:** Small adjustments may be the best course of action if a weakened posture is causing throat pain. This could be rearranging the keyboard, monitor, and seat at your workstation to create a more natural alignment for your head, neck, and body, or it could involve learning how to rest on your trunk with an ergonomic mattress and cushion rather than your stomach or other parts of your body.

- *Change your lifestyle:* If particular activities are shown to be the source of recurring throat pain, they may need to be avoided or curtailed. For example, if an individual typically uses their throat craned more for texting friends and looking at improvements than they should spend a few hours each day doing so, then that activity should be decreased; the phone should be positioned closer to the level of vision in order to keep the throat more carefully upright while texting.

- *Over-the-counter drugs:* A lot of over-the-counter analgesics have been shown to either minimize edema or prevent pain signals from reaching the brain. These medications can be utilized, but only very carefully. Read the directions and warnings on the entire label of the pain medicine, and take care not to take more than what is prescribed. For example, acetaminophen, the active ingredient in Tylenol, is also included in a wide range of other common medications, including those for colds and allergic reactions.

Alternative Medical Treatment for Throat Pain

For certain kinds of neck discomfort, medical management usually begins with non-surgical methods like you or a combination of the following:

- *Physical therapy:* To increase neck strength and adaptability, physical therapy is typically incorporated into most treatment plans. The structure and duration of the physical therapy program will vary based on the particular disease and circumstance. After attending several weekly lessons with a skilled physical therapist, the patient will eventually become proficient at performing the prescribed exercises at home.

- *Prescription analgesics:* Prescription-strength pain

relievers can be tried if over-the-counter options haven't worked. There are numerous painkillers available, and each one has advantages and disadvantages. Although the CDC changed its recommendations in 2016 and recommended less opioid prescriptions for the treatment of chronic pain, it was still generally recommended to use opioids due to the danger of addiction and other potential issues.

- Injections of cortisone steroid solution into the cervical epidural space—the outer layer of the spinal canal—are the procedure known as cervical epidural steroid injections. X-ray assistance (fluoroscopy) can be utilized to ensure that the injection switches into the epidural space adjacent to the inflamed nerve. The injection is intended to reduce nerve irritation or minimize the impact of a disc herniation on nearby tissues. These injections might lessen discomfort, enabling the patient to resume normal activities and make progress with a physical treatment regimen. This injection has certain risks, such as the possibility of infection, and its usage may only be permitted a few times year. It is also not always helpful.

- *Cervical facet injections:* Steroid injections into the appropriate bones might lessen pain if the discomfort in the facet crucial joints is the cause of the throat pain. Sometimes Radiofrequency Ablation (RFA) of the small sensory nerves that flow directly to the damaged facet crucial joints may be recommended if facet shots result in predictable but temporary relief. Although these RFA techniques might have more lasting effects, the purpose of these injections is to provide temporary relief for irritated facet bones rather than to solve the issue.

- *Trigger point shots:* Pain may be elicited by discomfort in particular muscle bundles. In order to restore the normal direction of the irritated muscle bundles, trigger point injections are used. Other than saline, lidocaine, dextrose, or cortisone, the injectable ingredients could be different. This kind of therapy may be subtle yet effective for throat muscle activation point irritations that are clearly identified. It's possible that these therapies won't be effective over the long run or won't reduce pain sufficiently.

- *Manual manipulation:* To increase flexibility and reduce pain, a chiropractor or other medical professional could manually adjust the spine. Usually performed on a desk in an office, manual manipulation is also referred to as a chiropractic adjustment. Usually, the chiropractor will adjust with his or her hands, but occasionally, little adjustments could be made with the use of a machine. While some claim that chiropractic realignment has lessened throat pain, not everyone is in favor of the procedure. High-velocity cervical backbone modifications have also been linked, albeit infrequently, to unfavorable outcomes like paralysis or heart attacks.

- *Acupuncture:* With roots in ancient Chinese medicine, acupuncture involves inserting tiny needles at certain points in the body, depending on the condition being treated. The average length of a treatment could be much less than an hour, including the removal of the needles. Needles in America are not meant to be reused; they must be disposed of. The acupuncturist's certification and usage of sterilized needles are crucial. Most patients tolerate acupuncture well, and it is generally regarded as safe.

Not all neck pain treatments are covered by the list above.

In addition to the aforementioned interventions, adopting a healthy lifestyle can also have a favorable effect on neck discomfort. For example, engaging in moderate aerobic exercise several times a week and quitting smoking can be beneficial for the majority of throat issues.

Chapter 8

Techniques for Relieving Throat Pain with Acupressure.

Back strain and muscle strain are frequently the causes of neck guitar pain. Divided cartilage and worn-out key joints could also be contributing factors. Usually, throat pain is concentrated in one area of the throat, although it can also spread. Tightness or spasms may be necessary to properly manage this kind of discomfort.

People have been using acupressure and reflexology for ages to treat neck pain. Acupressure locates points on the body that can be stimulated and rubbed to alleviate various ailments.

Reflexology's effectiveness in treating neck discomfort is still being studied, although anecdotal data suggests that it helps for many people. Learn more about the various factors that may help relieve your sore throat by reading on.

The Science of Neck Pain and Pressure Points

Many studies have been conducted on acupuncture, making it a reliable treatment for throat pain. Acupressure is not widely recognized as a treatment for throat pain because there is some evidence, Trusted Source, that acupuncture is effective in treating throat discomfort. For example, experts wonder if the acupuncture needles activate the same chemicals that heal. In such case, activating pressure factors using massage as opposed to needles wouldn't result in the same outcome.

That does not mean, however, that acupressure should no longer be used as a comprehensive treatment for throat pain. Reviving pressure variables have the potential to ease sore muscles and reduce throat pain. The answer is that individuals are ignorant, according to reviews of the medical texts conducted by multiple reliable sources.

Pressure Variables Associated with Throat Pain

To attempt treating your neck with acupressure, do the following:

- Unwind and take long breaths. Make sure the

space where the acupressure treatment is applied is suitable and peaceful.

- Apply firm, deep pressure to massage the pressure points that you have identified as being responsible for your sore throat. It is best to focus on each fingertip individually and spin them in a circular or up-and-down motion for three to four minutes at a time. If the treatment causes any sharpening or intensifying pain anywhere in your body, cease right away.

- If you think the therapeutic massage treatments are effective, repeat them throughout the day. The number of times a day that you can perform acupressure is unlimited.

A list of pressure locations for various kinds of throat pain is provided below. Recognize that the whole individual is interrelated in reflexology. This implies that stimulating one body area to activate or align another is a common occurrence.

The Jian Jing

Jian Jing is located in the neck muscles, midway between the starting point of your hands and the middle of your neck. This feature has been observed in reliable sources of muscle tension and successful acupuncture trials for headaches. Jian Jing could also be used to relieve sore throat or stiff throat pain. If you are pregnant, avoid encouraging this aspect to relieve your neck pain since it may trigger labor.

He Gu (L14)

The "web" fold of skin in the center of your thumb and fingers is where the He Gu point is located. According to reflexologists, activating this feature might lessen pain in your throat as well as many other parts of your body. Note: Do not revive this point if you are pregnant.

Pool of Blowing Wind (Feng Chi/GB20)

Feng Chi is located near the base of your skull, behind your earlobe, and towards the top of your throat. This indicates how reflexologists treat anything from headaches to tiredness. Applying pressure to this spot can help ease a sore throat brought on by an unpleasant sleeping position.

Zhong Zu (TE3)

The Zhong Zu point is located above your pinky and ring fingers, in the space between your knuckles. When this pressure point is stimulated, it may alleviate tension and encourage blood flow to different parts of the brain. In order to reduce pressure- or stress-related neck ache from playing the guitar, stimulate this area.

The Pillar of Heaven

This point is located at the base of your skull, on either side of your neck, and approximately two inches from the point where your backbone starts at its strongest. Just over your shoulder blades is where it is. Inflammated lymph nodes and congestion that might cause a sore neck may be released by stimulating this area Trusted Source.

Acupressure Elements for Neck Care

Employed Acupressure

Acupressure is a very useful treatment for pain in the

neck of the guitar and tightness in the throat. Acupressure points for treating the neck can be found all over the body. These days, throat pain and tightness are common issues. There are several ways to reduce throat pain and tightness, including medicine, acupuncture, acupressure, and more. This acupressure includes the simpler and superior method for treating throat pain.

Stress, tightness in the neck and shoulders, and a host of other pains can all be relieved using acupressure factors for neck pain. Acupressure Factors' primary feature is that it has no side effects. Using acupressure factors to treat guitar neck pain is completely safe. An age-old, risk-free method for treating throat pain is acupressure.

It takes only a few acupressure points to reduce discomfort and stop the decline or hit back. When used properly and frequently, acupressure factors are simple to employ and offer quicker relief from gout and glenohumeral joint pain. There are a number of acupressure points across the body, which go by the following names:

- Acupressure Elements for Neck Care.

- Acupressure Points on the Back of the Neck.

- Acupressure points on the head's back.

- Acupressure Points on the Back and Shoulders.

- Face Acupressure Factors.

Acupressure factors are helpful in relieving tightness and pain in the throat. These are the pressure factors that relate to throat pain:

- Neck Pain Acupressure Factors.

- Acupressure Points on the Back of the Neck.

Neck Backside Factors are helpful in relieving headache and throat pain. The rear of the throat contains six Acupressure Throat Backside Points in total. The three components of the Throat Backside Factors are the Heavenly Pillar, Windows of Heaven, and Gates of Awareness. Let's talk about each of the three sections separately:

The Awareness Gates:

The rear of your throat is home to Gates of Awareness points. In the space between your throat's muscles, locate the Acupressure Gates of Awareness Factors. The back muscles of the throat are perpendicular, and the pressure factors are located close to the base of the head. The Gates of Awareness are located, as depicted in the image.

At Gates of Consciousness, firm pressure applied to the nape of your neck can relieve headaches, dizziness, irritation, and stiff neck pain.

Reasons for Neck Pain with Acupressure

Heaven's home window is a crucial component of the Throat backside Points. Located beneath the Skull and near the Gates of Awareness, the Heaven Acupressure Factors for Throat Pain screen is situated in the rear of Throat. The exact location of Windows of Heaven Factors is on the base of the skull notch. Locate the Windowpane of Heaven Factors, as shown in the following image:

For optimal benefits, apply the appropriate pressure on Window of Heaven daily. If you routinely activate the Home Window of Heaven Factors, you can reduce headaches, neck pain, throat tightness, and glenohumeral joint pain.

As the Heavenly Pillar, Neck Backside Factors have two pressure factors. The Heavenly Pillar Factors are located beneath the skull's foot. The Heavenly Pillar Acupressure Factors are located precisely 2-3 millimeters below the base of the skull. Locate the pressure factors for the Heavenly Pillars, as indicated in the illustration, and apply pressure often with your hand or hands.

Regularly applying pressure to the Heavenly Pillar Acupressure Factors will help you reduce stress, fatigue, burnout, heavy thoughts, and other symptoms including sleeplessness and stiff neck. For neck pain and other neck-related issues, acupressure factors on the back of the neck should be stimulated in daily routine in order to achieve faster and more significant benefits.

Acupressure Elements on the Rear of the Mind:

It's important to remember the Back of Mind Point for Neck Pain. The exact rear of your mind is home to the Acupressure Back Again Mind Point. Wind Mansion is another name for the area behind Hands Point. The base of the skull is above THE TRUNK of Head Point. Locate the Acupressure Back of Mind Point, as indicated by the illustration below:

You can lessen neck pain, eyes-ear pain, nasal pain, stiff neck, throat issues, make pain, and other pains by regularly applying firm pressure to the top point of the acupressure triangle.

Elements of Acupressure for the Shoulder Back:

Factors related to the shoulders and back are very helpful in reducing tension and pain. The location of the acupressure shoulder back factors is not on the lower neck, but rather on the glenohumeral joint collection 3 centimeters. Make WellPoint is another name for the glenohumeral joint back yet point. To prevent issues, locate the exact location of the Acupressure Glenohumeral joint Back Still Point and apply light pressure. The following is a picture of Make Back Factors:

- You can get relief from a variety of symptoms, including weariness, irritability, glenohumeral joint stress, and make pain, by routinely applying the appropriate pressure on acupressure glenohumeral joint back factors.

- Extreme caution: If a person is pregnant, please refrain from applying any pressure to the back factors of the glenohumeral joint.

Acupuncture Elements for the Face

Spa and therapeutic massage:

Face Factors are the best treatment for sore throats. The acupressure face factors for throat pain are located on the nasal bridge, just below the ends of the eyebrows. Bamboo Drilling Factors for Throat Pain is also mentioned. The exact location of Face Point is where the brow's end and the nasal bridge meet. The following picture illustrates the Acupressure Face Factors for

Throat Pain:

To treat conditions like headaches, sinuses, hay fever, and neck pain, apply pressure on the Acupressure Face Factors for Neck Pain every day.

Commonly accessible acupressure points:

Hand factors provide relief from sore throats and tight throats. Two distinct locations on the hands correspond to the Acupressure Hand Factors for Throat Pain. The index and middle fingers are home to the first hands point. Start by referring to the image below to determine First Hands Point's precise location. To advance results and relieve neck tightness and throat pain, gently press the First Hands Point during daily activities.

The location of the Second Hands Point for Throat Pain is near the final little finger (pinky). The Acupressure Point is positioned specifically beneath the little finger. Locate the pressure point as indicated by the illustration below. Put firm pressure on the Hands Indicate to relieve your sore throat.

The Top 6 Acupressure Points to Treat Pain in the Throat

The throat, located slightly below the top, is a very important bodily component. Although the brain is located in the mind, the throat has the ability to change the brain in any way it pleases. But because of modern technology and our computer-dependent lifestyle, we experience aches and pains more frequently, including pain in the throat and other areas, which is also typically the cause of excruciating headaches. Reflexology can be used to effectively provide long-term relief from distress and unpleasant sensations in the top and throat areas. These points are all yang components with intense energy circulation.

Acupressure Elements for the Management of Glenohumeral Joint and Throat Pain

Factors contributing to pharyngitis:

There are many different causes of neck and shoulder pain and stiffness, ranging from absurd ones like sleeping in the wrong position to more serious ones like arthritis and meningitis, which can leave us with a hurting and aching neck for several days.

massage of the neck

The following are a few typical causes of guitar neck pain:

- Bad Posture While Seated.

- Bad alignment when sleeping.

- Strain in the muscles.

- Excessive effort.

- Pour.

- Pain in the neck.

In all cases, it is typical to have discomfort ranging from dull aches to numbness in the neck and shoulder area. These symptoms usually go away in a few days with easy workouts. On the other hand, there are situations where the tightness in the throat can last for several weeks or even months, accompanied by shoulder blades, the back, and even a headache.

Among the major causes of shoulder and neck pain are:

- **Meningitis:** Enlargement of the meninges around the brain.

- **Arthritis:** Rheumatoid arthritis and cervical spondylitis.

In such instances, professionals must provide emergency medical help.

Using Acupressure to Reduce Pain and Aches in the Shoulders and Throat

Although glenohumeral joint and neck problems can be highly dangerous and interfere with our daily activities, reflexology can heal these conditions from the inside out, leading to total body and mind peace instead of turning to temporary fixes like painkillers.

The Top 6 Acupressure Points for Shoulder and Neck Pain Relief

Acupuncture is a comprehensive healing method that has

its roots in traditional eastern healing arts. It helps treat both the mild and bothersome aches and pains as well as the chronic, throbbing aches and pains that are a common occurrence in modern life. It can support us in regaining our sense of equilibrium and lowering tension. To relieve discomfort and tightness in the throat and shoulder, you can use these six basic acupressure elements on yourself or get someone you care about enrolled in a restorative acupressure program.

Region of the Shoulders:

Shoulder region: This area is located on the biceps muscle, halfway between the foot of the neck and the glenohumeral joint's end. In order to relieve shoulder and throat tightness, this component might be stimulated. Additionally, it helps to relieve back pain.

Area Around the Eyes:

Completion Bone: This part is located in the SCM muscle's dip behind the hearing on the occipital crest. Reviving this point helps to relieve dizziness, headache, and throat pain.

Neck Area:

Heaven's Pillar: This feature is located on the occipital ridge, directly next to the tendon where the backbone enters the skull. Rousing this spot helps to relieve tightness in the neck, numbness, and discomfort. Reviving this area also aids in the reduction of persistent cough.

Principal Region:

There are about seven points in another location that are at the top. With the aid of figures 1 through 7, we have illustrated these elements in the diagram, starting with the forehead. Combining all of these elements at once helps to relieve frontal headaches and neck pain brought on by arthritis.

Region of the Side Throat:

The celestial region is located in the muscle, beneath and to the slight back of the earlobe. Reviving this point helps ease headaches, tension in the shoulders and throat, and headaches.

Hands:

Union Valley: This feature is located in the web that runs between your index and thumb fingers. Raising this point helps ease tension and apprehension in the shoulders and throat. Reviving this element is also a good method to reduce tension and anxiety.

Eight Easy Steps to a Fruitful Acupressure Session:

- Now that you are aware of the specific acupressure sites that can be stimulated to reduce throat pain and improve the area, here are a few easy suggestions you can use to help the recipient have an amazing experience with the program.

- Acquire a clear understanding of the receiver's trouble area.

- Prior to starting the acupressure session, ask the recipient to perform a couple stretches.

- Assign the recipient to lie down on the spotless mat.

- Keep supplies close at reach, such as pillows and towels.

- Place clean cloths or wrapped towels for support anyplace on your body that does not come into touch with the mat.

- Start by gently pressing the factors with your fingertips, and ask the person if the pressure feels wonderful.

- At the same time, apply pressure to the same areas on both sides of your body.

- Press on a particular area for two to three minutes before moving on to another spot.

Acupressure has a long history and has been successfully used to treat a wide range of conditions for a very long time. Experience the soothing effects of the intense therapy as it permeates your being and replenishes the natural elements and the entire amount in the middle of your body. Don't forget to discuss how reflexology can help with neck pain.

Chapter 9

Pain Management Using Trapezium

There are trigger points in the trapezius that are frequently present. Patients visit an office more frequently for referred pain resulting from these trigger points than for almost any other issue. The image illustrates the large kite-shaped muscle known as the trapezius, which covers a large portion of the posterior pharynx and trunk. The muscle is divided into three primary regions: the top, middle, and lower trapezius. Each region has unique functions and symptoms related to the joints.

Usual Indications of Trapezium Discomfort

Freeze glenohumeral joint workouts contain myofascial trigger elements.

Superior Trapezius

- temple headaches, often known as "pressure" headaches

- Jaw, cheek, or temple pain

- Anguish concealed by attentiveness

- vertigo or dizziness (related to the sternocleidomastoid muscle)

- excruciating neck pain

- A tense neck

- restricted range of mobility

- An intolerance for carrying a lot of weight.

Trapezius in the middle

- One mid-back ache

- Pain in the base of your skull two

- A trigger point is a localized area of searing pain that is close to the spine.

- Trigger point 6 connects painful sensations to the shoulder's superior aspect, near joint 3.

Trapezius Lower

- Pain in the upper back, throat, or midback 4

- Similar to the stratus posterior superior referral pattern, there may be a referral on the shoulder blade's trunk, down the inside of the arm, and into the ring and little fingers (Trigger point 7).

- Pain in the base of the skull

- Deep pain and spreading discomfort outrageous of the glenohumeral joint might be referred to as trigger point 3.

- Trapezius: Activate Point Images

- Use point therapy while exercising to treat an icy shoulder at home by freezing

- Tendinitis and rotator cuff muscle workouts.

Reasons for Induce Points and Their Continuence

- A limb that is shorter than the other

- A smaller hemipelvis employing only one portion (the section of the pelvis you sit on)

- Short upper arms (which forces you to slenderize to one side in order to use the armrests)

- Big breasts

- drowsiness

- ☐ Stiffening your upper body

- Holding a phone between your shoulder and middle ear

- A seat with insufficient or excessive armrests

- Overusing a keyboard to type

- Stitching while keeping your hands unsupported on your lap

- Running

- Sleeping with your head turned away for a long time when lying on your front or back

- Taking up the violin

- Athletics characterized by abrupt, unilateral

motions

- drooping or not firmly leaning against a support when sitting

- Traveling by foot

- Riding a bike

- Canoeing

Any profession or activity that necessitates extended periods of flexion, such as electronic work, dentistry or hygienic work, architectural or sketch work, and secretarial or computer work

- Overly tight bra straps, whether on the band or the torso strap

- An overstuffed purse or daypack

- An ill-fitting, thick layer

No matter how light your pack or backpack may seem, you are still hiking up one make when you carry it over one glenohumeral joint every day.

Whiplash can result from a quick movement of the top, a car accident, or landing on your mind.

- Projective stance

- Using a cane while walking takes too much time.

- Selecting a single section of your account to engage in conversation for extended periods of time

- Pectoralis major muscles are restricted.

Practical Hints

See a professional to obtain padding or raises that compensate for any asymmetry in your upper arms or body. Make adjustments or replace any mismatched furniture. The seat needs to be close enough so that you may lower fat against your backrest and your legs should be able to fit under the table. Either on your project surface or on the armrests at the same height, your elbows should be comfortable. On the armrests, your forearms and elbows should rest equally. When you can, you should be able to stare straight ahead at your computer screen, with the replica situated on the medial side of the screen.

A slanted work surface will reduce the mechanical strain to a spot if you must lean over to examine documents or programs (such as an architect, engineer, or draftsman), but remember to take regular rests.

Invest in a speaker or headset for your phone, or use one hand to hold the phone. The shoulder rests are insufficient. Put on bras that fit properly. The straps are too tight if, after removing your bra, you can see elastic marks on your skin. For women with medium or small breasts, running bras are perfect. Ask the salesman to help you choose a bra that fits well; the majority of them are knowledgeable about their merchandise.

Get rid of any foam rubber cushions you may have! These pillows' vibrations will exacerbate some outcomes. If you are lying down, your cushion should support your head at a rate that is comfortable for you—not too much or too little. When I travel, I usually bring my cushion with me. I am aware that I have a cozy place to slumber, and that it will be useful if I ever get stuck at an airport.

Should your doctor recommend breast reduction surgery, your insurance company might pay for it if your breasts are so big that they give you backaches. If you are considering surgery, give it serious thought and weigh the dangers.

Put your daypack on top of both shoulders. If you plan to bring a handbag, choose one with an elongated strap so you can wear the belt over your head, positioning it diagonally across your torso. The material should also be light.

Try to balance the majority of your weight on your hip strap if you are wearing a backpack. Since head-forward posture can both generate and perpetuate trigger points, correct position restoration, particularly with regard to head location, is essential to treating contributing variables. Seated in front of a computer, at a table, while eating dinner, or while watching television can all exacerbate a head-forward position. You may correct weak sitting position by using superb lumbar support practically anywhere you sit.18 To begin postural re-training, watch the video below.

Take frequent breaks if you must sit for extended amounts of time. Setting a timer for the room will ensure that you have to get up quickly to safely turn it off.

When engaging in a conversation, turn to face the other person instead of turning your thoughts toward them. When standing up, the trapezius muscle must bear the weight of your hands in your pockets. The glenohumeral joint cushions can be layered to alleviate some of the higher trapezius's pressure.

In order to rule out occipital neuralgia and cerviocogenic headaches, you might wish to consult a medical professional if activate point self-help measures aren't working for you. You might want to get checked for misaligned vertebrae by an osteopathic physician or chiropractor.

Techniques for Self-Help

On the CD-ROM, general suggestions for applying these

self-help methods are covered in detail. To place an order, simply click this link. Please be advised that if you do not follow the exact advice as presented on the CD-ROM, you may exacerbate the discomfort.

Putting Pressure on

Lay faceup with your legs bent on a firm bed or the floor. Start at the make, about one in and out from the backbone, and maintain pressure for eight seconds to a minute per spot with a golf ball or racquetball. Move a little bit further down the trunk to a new location, and keep moving gradually to maintain pressure on each place. Continue until you can get beneath the rib cage (the video shows you going all the way to the top of the pelvis, but you only need to go underneath the rib cage for the trapezius). If you have a wide back or soft factors farther out, you may want to carry on with this on another line farther right out of the spine. Generally, avoid doing this to the spine!

Lay your forearm and elbow on the surface at a height that will support the weight of your equipment. Using your opposing hand, bend your head slightly to the side you'll be working on, reach across your front, and pinch the upper portion of your trapezius muscle. Don't press your thumb into the indentation above the collar bone; instead, stay on the tissue's meat.

The upper trapezius will also be treated by the supraspinatus muscle self-help. Place a rugby ball in the doorjamb groove while standing in a doorway, then steadily store the ball with your other hand. As you bend at a 90-degree angle, make sure your mind goes entirely limp! Choose your desired level of pressure and slim into the ball. Work places all over the shoulder, maintaining the ball in your other hand and continuing to maintain complete mental composure.

Use a baseball and place your hands behind your neck, face up, to concentrate on the trunk of your neck. With the baseball in the center of the best palm—not where the fingers sign up for the palm—one palm should be directly on top of the other. Rotate your thoughts toward the ball to apply pressure (don't place the ball on your back; instead, use the muscles that aren't attached to your spine). To move the ball, turn your head away from the medial side you plan to focus on, rotate your mind back toward the medial side you plan to work on, and then move the ball a little bit. Turn your account to the medial side that you will work on even more if you want greater pressure, and rotate your mindless if you want less pressure. Generally speaking, don't decide to attend to the ball! The muscles may feel more pressure as a result of this. Make sure you turn your head away from the ball in order to move it. Work down the base of the head, down the neck's trunk, and try to reach all the way to the base of the throat where it meets the finest part of the glenohumeral joint.

Workouts

Swimming is a great cardio workout that doesn't put a lot of strain on your muscles. Make sure to vary the way you stroke so as not to overstress the trapezius.

- Concentrating on a one area can exacerbate the trapezius, much like a crawl heart attack.

- Continue while leaping rope.

Place your hands at your sides and point your thumbs forward while standing with your feet about four inches apart. To stabilize your back, tighten your buttocks. Then, while breathing in, twist your hands and shoulder blades back and forth (turning your thumbs back), pressing your neck into the trunk. As you continue to hold this posture and release your breath, lower your shoulder blades. Take a deep breath in and out normally while you bring your mind back to align your hearing with your shoulder blades. Hold this position for around six seconds. After releasing the present, relax, but try to hold your posture correctly (do not open your lips or move your nose while moving your mind). If you find that maintaining this posture is uncomfortable or too "stiff," consider shifting your weight from your pumps to the balls of your feet, which will push your head back between your shoulder blades. At least once every hour to two hours, you should perform this exercise repeatedly throughout the day to help you retrain your posture. Performing one repetition six times or more a day is preferable to performing six repetitions consecutively.

Trapezius trigger factors are quite prevalent and have been linked to numerous conditions, including stiff necks and headaches. One important muscle that moves the make is the trapezius. The top fibers help to prevent the glenohumeral joint girdle from depressing during weight transfer by pulling it upward.

The upper and bottom trapezius muscles generate trigger factors. The majority of us maintain our top trigger points, which are usually tied to our positions and are usually active.

Numerous common ailments, such as chronic tension and neck pain, whiplash, stress headaches, cluster headaches, cervical backbone pain, face/jaw pain, neck pain and stiffness, top glenohumeral joint discomfort, mid-back pain, and dizziness, are linked to these trigger variables.

The good news is that trigger points in the upper trapezius are very easily accessed, and there are numerous at-home exercises you may perform on your own to assist release these "knots" in order to receive treatment and, in certain cases, achieve more flexibility in the shoulders and neck.

Technique for Trigger Point Personal Therapy

The goal of this approach is to locate the trigger's or tender point's core. This might cause a mostly known pain map to be triggered when squeezed, ideally replicating your experiences.

This method entails exerting consistent, mild, and direct pressure on the concept.

Methods

Determine the delicate areas that you plan to address.

Assign the sponsor muscle to a comfortable, fully extended position that allows it to relax.

Once resistance is felt, gently apply pressure on the soft point and increase it gradually. Rather than being felt as pain, this will be perceived as soreness.

Maintain pressure on the sensitive area until you feel it produce and soften. This could take a few seconds to many minutes.

You can go back and repeat steps 3–4 until the soft or trigger point totally yields. The strain is gradually increased.

You might try to improve the pressure of these repetitions' journey to get a better outcome. Take great caution and always use common sense!

You probably have trigger points for a variety of reasons, so it's important to consider how your trigger point discomfort relates to other body parts. It is important to emphasize that the methods provided on this website are not a substitute for professional therapy.

Trigger point aches and pains are understandable, however there may frequently be an underlying pathology.

It is advised to get an official diagnosis from a properly qualified specialist at all times. Use a buddy or partner if at all possible; see the above procedure notes for details.

Individualized Care Using Fingertips

It's definitely a good idea to start feeling the activate

point itself with your fingertips (fingertips) rather than just the nearby area. A variety of pressure instruments are available for purchase. They invite you to simply reach a potential neighborhood and are reasonably priced. We think that every person ought to have a pressure tool!

Stretching by itself is unlikely to significantly reduce the induce points, but it may be very helpful in treating them and, when combined with self-care, can hasten the healing process.

Always begin cautiously and proceed with utmost caution. If the agony becomes too great, stop. Before you expand, get professional guidance if you already have a painful issue.

Self-directed care

Research has consistently demonstrated the significance and worth of self-managed care. It's amazing how easy it can be to get treatment when using basic methods like the ones mentioned above.

Whenever you suffer from chronic or long-term pain

conditions, it is usually useful to work with a qualified specialist.

The majority of therapists can assist you in creating a self-managed treatment plan and may even be able to teach you the proper use of pressure instruments.

The Trapezius Muscle's Anatomy

One of the main problems in the spine and on either side of the spine is the trapezius muscle. Stretching from the occipital bone of the skull to the inferior thoracic vertebrae of the backbone, it is regarded as a vast surface muscle. The scapula, or make blade, is moved, rotated, and stabilized by the trapezius muscle.

There are three rings of muscle fibers that make up the trapezius muscle, and each has its own unique structure and purpose. They all collaborate with one another. They facilitate the movement of the backbone and the glenohumeral joint blade.

Superior fibers: Located on the lateral and posterior neck margins, these fibers lift the make blade, enabling motions similar to a shrug for all of us.

- Middle fibers: Found extending into the acromion process of the scapula along the superior thoracic vertebrae. The glenohumeral joint blade is pulled closer to the spine by the center fibers through its adduction and retractions.

- Inferior fibers: Covers a wide area of the trunk stem, extending from the inferior thoracic vertebrae to the scapula spine. By drawing the shoulder blade closer to the weak thoracic vertebrae, the second-rate fibers depress the shoulder blade.

What May Induce Pain in the Trapezius Muscle?

• *Pulling muscles:* This happens when a tissue is moved too quickly or excessively, which can cause harm. Your muscles may become less mobile and cause pain as a result of the severing of their connections.

- *Stress:* When a person is overcome with fear, their muscles, especially their trapezius muscles, may tense up or become worried. That is mainly brought on by greater tightening of the muscles, which causes soreness and pain. Stress, both mental and physical, can exacerbate these symptoms and are frequently associated with stressful times.

- *Poor posture:* In addition to various issues involving the vertebral vertebrae and supporting muscles, sitting or being positioned incorrectly can cause pain in the trapezius muscle. If the incorrect circumstance is not addressed quickly, it may become irreversible.

- *Pressure:* Excessive or restricted strain on the trapezius can cause the muscle to become stressed, which can cause pain. Wearing bulky backpacks, creating purses, or even having restricted bra straps might cause this.

- *Holding positions:* Maintaining uncomfortable sitting or standing postures can cause pain in the trapezius muscle. Another name for this may be repeated stress injury.

- ***Traumatic injury:*** Severe injuries like whiplash or direct head trauma can cause pain in the trapezius muscle. A forceful snapping back and forth in your head puts strain on your trapezius muscle.

Making A Trapezius Strain Diagnosis

A medical professional who treats your undiagnosed trapezius strain will ask you detailed questions about where and why you are experiencing discomfort, as well as why it is becoming better and worse. This greatly improves the doctor's ability to pinpoint the possible location of the pain. To rule out any underlying causes, a brief medical history and a list of medications may also be obtained.

The most common cause of a trapezius strain is an injury of some kind, therefore it's crucial to let your doctor know if you engage in any sports or perform any tasks at work that might have contributed to your symptoms of trapezius muscle pain.

The physical examination would come next. After examining the area to check for any signs of spine bruising, your doctor may ask you to move your hands and shoulder blades to demonstrate how the trapezius muscle discomfort is caused and which areas of the spine are sore and tense. Additional tests will analyze cerebral neuronal function, which includes a pinprick and light touch sensations. Reflexes are extended by the muscle, and power testing can also be quantified.

Certain procedures, like an MRI, are not necessary if the growing pain in the neck and shoulders is not accompanied by other indications or symptoms of the underlying illness.

Pain Management for Trapezius Muscle

- **_Calm down:_** Stressing out your muscles too much will interfere with their ability to heal. Pain from musculoskeletal disorders may get worse if you don't try to relax.

- **•_Ice:_** The application of snow to the affected area can effectively reduce pain and inflammation.

While a glaciers pack is the best option, frozen vegetables in a handbag or ice wrapped in a towel would also work perfectly. Every two to four hours, it is highly advised to snow the body part that is afflicted for 15 to 20 minutes.

- ***Heat Therapy:*** Using a warm towel or a hot shower can effectively relieve muscle tension. If you are very sensitive to temperature fluctuations, this may also extend to wearing warm clothing during the colder months. Moreover, warmth helps lessen discomfort and hasten the healing process. You can also utilize temperature packs, which you can make yourself or get already. Simply fill a small sock or pouch with rice and microwave it for two minutes.

- ***Epsom salts:*** Frequently used to warm baths, Epsom salts have the added benefit of relieving muscular aches. Its high magnesium concentration, which supports the remaining muscles and aches and pains, is the reason for this. For optimal outcomes, incorporate one or two cups of Epsom salts into your shower and immerse the afflicted area or entire body for a minimum of thirty minutes. Baths should be considered as often as three times a week till the strained muscle heals.

- **_Customizing Activities:_** Limiting physically demanding activities and making time for adequate rest can be beneficial. It can assist to relieve symptoms to know how to maintain a better posture, such as sitting at a table with your back to the chair or taking frequent breaks from sitting. A great rule of thumb is to make sure that, when sitting or standing upright, you can pass your hands through the lower gap.

- **_Pain Relief:_** Using non-steroidal anti-inflammatory medicines (NSAIDs) is a helpful supplement that can help reduce pain and inflammation even more. Ibuprofen (Motrin, Advil), naproxen (Aleve), and numerous additional prescription-only NSAIDs are examples of conventional NSAIDs. Using these medications requires following the doctor's instructions, and in addition, adverse effects are possible.

Massage to Reduce Pain in the Trapezius Muscle

Strains to the trapezius muscle may cause unpleasant knots or trigger points to form, which can cause pain and discomfort but is easily treated with pressure through massage. It is always advised to do massages with a clear view and to never apply too much pressure. The shoulder blades, the guitar neck, and the thoracic vertebral regions should be areas of focus. Some therapeutic massage techniques that you can try right now are listed below:

- *Tennis ball:* You can roll a firm object, like a golf ball, back and forth between your trapezius and a sensitive surface, such the ground. This type of massage focuses on the area that hurts.

- *Setting up:* You can help relax the trapezius muscle just by lying down. To support your throat and maintain it in line with your backbone, it is highly advised that you maintain a cushion beneath your thoughts. You could even extend your hand back and use your fingertips to massage the aching spot.

- **_Use a therapeutic massage tool:_** You may find a variety of devices and tools to help you reach difficult-to-reach places, such as the trunk. For a therapeutic massage for your trapezius muscle pain, you may opt for an electric method, but manual methods will also be beneficial.

Exercises for Straining the Trapezius Muscle

The trapezius can be stretched and worked, much like other thoracic muscles, to help reduce discomfort and tension. Some of the best exercises for treating discomfort in the trapezius muscle are listed below:

- **_Glenohumeral joint shrug:_** This exercise, which involves merely raising your shoulder blades toward your ear, tightening, and then releasing them, is thought to be among the best for relieving discomfort in the trapezius muscle. For an added stretch, you can even hold dumbbells in each hand.

- **_Right rows:_** To begin, stand with your foot

shoulder-width apart. Place a set of dumbbells in front of your thighs and press them there. Raise the dumbbells in front of you to the level of your glenohumeral joint and then carefully lower them back down.

- **_Shoulder movement:_** Once again, maintain a straight back and a shoulder-width apart. Then, begin to raise your shoulder blades upward and forth in a circular motion. Rotation needs to be controlled and done slowly. This exercise can even be done backwards.

- **_Yoga neck extends:_** Stand upright with your feet shoulder-width apart and your arms at your sides. Raise your right arm and gradually tilt your head to the left until you feel an extension. Now repeat on the other side. After finishing both edges, softly push forward with both hands on the trunk of your mind until you feel an extension in your throat and down your chest. Before releasing, hold each extension for about 20 to 30 milliseconds.

Chapter 10

Scalene

The scalene consists of the scalenus anterior, scalenus medius, and scalenus posterior, three pairs of muscles in the lateral pharynx. The scalenus minimus, a fourth muscle, can occasionally be seen behind the lower portion of the scalenus anterior. Between your anterior and middle scalenes, the brachial plexus and subclavian artery come together. The subclavian vein and phrenic nerve travel anteriorly to the anterior scalene, crossing the first rib.

Placement

- The ascending cervical artery, which supplies blood to all three of your scalenus muscle divisions, is a branch of the thyro-cervical trunk.

Action: Rotates and flexes the neck

Function: In addition to flexing and laterally bending the neck to the same side, the anterior and middle scalene muscles lift the first rib. The posterior scalene's function is to raise the following bone and incline the neck toward the same side. They also develop into auxiliary inspiration muscles in conjunction with the sternocleidomastoid.

Diseases:

Regional pain symptoms known as scalene myofascial pain symptoms occur when pain starts in the throat region and travels down. This issue may arise as a secondary or major cause of basic cervical disease. A significant number of problems involving chest muscular pain are related to induce point activity in the Scalene muscle group. In order to effectively treat their clients' complaints of upper body pain, spine pain, glenohumeral joint pain, radiating equip pain or thoracic store symptoms, wrist pain, and hand pain, therapists must have an in-depth understanding of this muscle group and its trigger points.

These trigger points can result in upper body pain as well as difficulty breathing in and out; many customers worry greatly that they may be having heart symptoms.

Thoracic outlet syndrome is one clinical diagnosis that these muscle sensations may be related to.

- Tendinitis of the subacromials.

- Tendinitis in the bistitium.

- Epicondylitis of the left leg.

- Torticollis spasmodic (symptoms of wryneck).

- Syndrome of carpal tunnel.

- Cervical rib syndrome, or costoclavicular syndrome

Whiplash injuries are one activity that can result in discomfort and pain in the scalene.

- Prolonged coughing.

- Gasping for air (those with bronchitis, pneumonia, emphysema, or asthma are particularly susceptible to issues with their scalene muscles).

- Grasping or pulling with hands at waist level.

- Working for extended periods of time while viewing the mind as a single entity ("word-processor headaches").

- Dozing on your stomach while focusing only on one side of your thoughts.

- Bringing a large purse or backpack.

- Donning an appropriate collar or harness.

Check for Scalene

- *Individual Position:* A typical person would lie supine with their hands raised above their heads and their head rotated to the contralateral aspect that has to be evaluated.

- *Position of Specialist:* The specialist stands at the top of the desk, placing their fingertips on the typical person's forehead.

- *Definition of Muscle Test:* An average individual is asked to flex their upper body against a mild resistance set by the practitioner.

Therapy:

The first action you need to take to get rid of your scalene Eliminating trigger points entails addressing the root issues.

Gently press the tips of your right hand's fingers against the other side of your neck. Apply little pressure to a discreet area of the throat. Repeat to both sides and in a little different area of the throat. Please repeat the motion five to ten times on either side of the throat.

Before performing this exercise, it may be helpful to place a hot pack or heating pad over the throat for ten to twenty-five minutes. Use appropriate diaphragmatic breathing in and out between extends. Breathe deeply and slowly to help relax your throat. Place the hands of the medial side that needs to be stretched under your buttocks in order to lower and anchor its shape. Put the other hand above your head, meaning that your fingertips should be speaking to the best part of your ear.

Stretch the medial side of your neck by gently pulling the top and neck to the opposite side, releasing the tension in your neck muscles as needed. Try to bring your ear all the way down to your shoulder.

You will now rotate your thoughts, and the scalene that is targeted will depend on how much you rotate. Move that person toward the equipment that is tugging in order to concentrate on the posterior scalene.

Turn your face away from the pulling provide in order to concentrate on the anterior scalene. Look straight up at the roof, or just a little bit in the direction of the pulling arm, to aim the center scalene.

When you swivel your head to focus on a particular muscle, concentrate all of your attention and energy on that muscle that appears to be the tightest. For approximately six to seven seconds, hold the stretches.

Scalene settles into a cozy chair to power. Put your right hand's palm on the right side of your brain. In the activity, this hand serves as a stabilizing hand. Maintaining the degree of resistance supplied by your right hands, begin to move your correct hearing in the direction of your right glenohumeral joint. Repeat each step eight to twelve times. You can lessen the likelihood of repeat injury by strengthening your cervical backbone through scalene muscle conditioning.

Sit or work directly while listening to a resistance music group looped in your head as an additional scalene exercise. Make sure there is definitely some pressure inside the music group by keeping the ends firmly to one side. With your mind still in its normal state, resist the want to move the music group away from you. Maintain this stance, unwind, and repeat.

Acknowledgements

Behold the magnificent triumph of this extraordinary book, a testament to the divine intervention of God Almighty and the unwavering love and support of my cherished Family, devoted Fans, avid Readers, loyal Customers, and dear Friends. Their ceaseless encouragement has paved the way for this resounding success.

www.ingramcontent.com/pod-product-compliance
Lightning Source LLC
Chambersburg PA
CBHW031126020426
42333CB00012B/259